NATURAL HAIR FOR BEGINNERS

A BEGINNER'S GUIDE TO GOING NATURAL SUCCESSFULLY!

SABRINA R PERKINS

CONTENTS

INTRODUCTION

Hello to all women of color who choose to relinquish the hold of chemicals on their hair and bodies, and embrace going natural! This book is for all women who want or need to take a more natural approach to their haircare, and I am thrilled to be sharing this step- by-step method. Natural Hair For Beginners was created to share my 11+ years of experience with going natural and discussing every step along the way.

I created this book because I saw there was a real need for a comprehensive tool for any woman who wants to go natural and do it successfully. From products to styling to ingredients, this book gives all the pertinent information you will need to not only go natural but to STAY natural. You learn what natural oils are best for hair growth, what constitutes as a protective style and how to grow your hair to longer lengths faster. I've included EVERYTHING!

Many women fail at going natural because there is no place to find all the information needed to leave relaxers alone for good. Now, you have what you need! I know this book will be a real asset to your natural hair journey. Every chapter gives in-depth guidance on what natural hair is, offers the do and don'ts, and answers every natural hair question you could ever have.

NOTE TO THE READER

Hello future Naturalistas! Sabrina here! Just wanting to thank you for buying the book and taking the plunge into natural hair living. Yes, it's a lifestyle change and one for the better. I truly hope this book brings you all the knowledge, support and guidance necessary for a successful natural hair journey. As you read the book, keep in mind that this is your own personal journey and different from anyone else's. So, enjoy the ride!

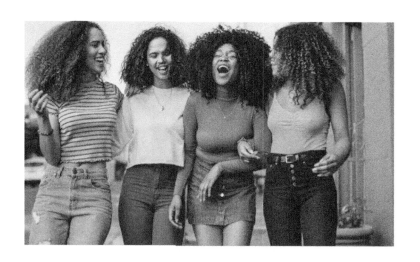

CHAPTER ONE

WHAT IS NATURAL HAIR & AM I READY TO "GO NATURAL?"

Once upon a time there was a black girl who thought a pressing comb and/or a perm were her only hair options. My, how far we have come since then! As the Natural Hair Revolution has taken hold within the last decade, black and brown women have been exploring the new options of rocking their own natural texture instead of relying on straightening techniques like hot combs, flat irons or relaxer creams. To a woman who has been relaxed from the age 13 to 35, that sounds like a frightening yet, amazing liberation.

Once I began doing my own hair as a child, I knew of only one way to care for it and that was with relaxer creams. Now, we have options with our natural texture but, what exactly is a woman to do? What do I use and will my hair grow? For us to fully answer those questions, we need to know what we are dealing with and first off is to know what natural hair really is.

WHAT IS NATURAL HAIR?

In a nutshell, natural hair is the hair you are born with, that you leave unaltered by chemicals. When I say chemicals, I only mean those items that alter the makeup of your hair from one texture to another. We are not talking about hair coloring as most do not change your hair's texture; on the other hand, perms, relaxers and texturizers do.

Some even call us embracing our natural hair a "movement." Many even flag a rejection of the European style of beauty, especially on hair type and texture. Natural hair is a closing of assimilation and an opening of self-appreciation. Too deep? Well, for the hundreds of women who go natural every week, all that is true. While some may see it merely as a hairstyle change, if one is to go natural successfully, the action of going natural is deeper than just wanting to try a new trend.

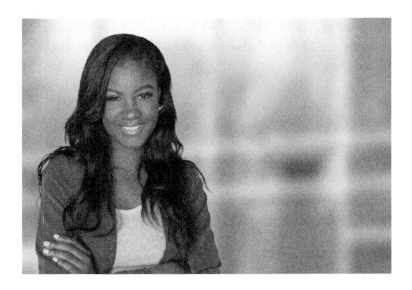

AM I READY TO "GO NATURAL?"

I, unfortunately, did not have the luxury of asking myself this question. Back in 2005, we had moved from a humid climate to a dry one. With such a drastic change, I was unsure of how my hair would fare if I'd continued to use chemicals. So, I opted for going natural without KNOWING I was going natural. I simply stopped relaxing my hair. For three years, I rocked wigs and braids. Finally, after thinning edges and an annoyance of not seeing my own hair, I chopped off all my hair and rocked a Teeny-Weeny Afro. My natural hair journey had begun!

My going natural story may be very different from yours, but the desire to leave chemicals alone is probably similar. Back then, natural hair wasn't quite a thing or at least it wasn't in my orbit, so I had to scope out products and tips to care for my new do. In the beginning, it was pretty tragic. There were no product lines specifically designed for natural hair. Natural oils for hair were not realized in products and not many sources like blogs, magazines or even books were out to help. I was on my own and my hair suffered as a result. I suffered from dryness and breakage, and didn't know the mechanics of natural hair to give it what it needed.

Well, somehow, I prevailed and learned more about my hair and myself by simply removing relaxers from my vocabulary and life. My struggles do not need to be your struggles and going natural is much easier than it was eight years ago. Today, it is as simple as cutting off your hair or no longer relaxing.

Yes, there are tons of places to get information on natural hair but where is everything from A to Z? Nowhere, actually, and that's why I created this book. Not only will this book cover every area of healthy hair care, it will even let you know if you are ready willing and able to go natural.

SO, HOW DO YOU KNOW YOU ARE READY?

You are ready when you want to make a lifestyle change in your life, in regards to your hair. Yes, I said a lifestyle change. Going natural is not a fad or a new hairstyle to try for a few weeks or months. Rock a natural hair wig for adventure, but going natural means having an openness to relearn how to care for your hair, using different products, methods and tools and having a willingness to step outside of your comfort zone. Then and only then will you be ready and able to go natural. If you feel this is for you, then it's time to take the plunge and learn how to go natural the successful way!

CHAPTER TWO

HOW TO GO NATURAL: THE MOST IMPORTANT STEPS

Yes, there are particular steps to take in order to go natural. No, you do not have to adhere to a rigid system that may or may not work for you. This is your personal journey, but taking heed to particular tips while on that journey can be the difference between going natural successfully or going back to the creamy crack for the umpteenth time.

In no way am I implying it takes only a few steps to go natural with black hair, but there are vital steps to get the natural hair ball rolling. Going natural should and can be a freeing and positive experience, but many women have serious questions before they decide to take the plunge:

How do I go natural?

Is going natural hard?

Can just anybody go natural?

Unfortunately, there are just too few how-tos that give step-by-step directions on how to care for natural black hair. That is the main reason for this book! Yes, you can scour the web for articles and blogs that give fruitful information, but where can you get step 1 to 100? This is also the reason far too many women end up failing at this process. Some of us just need a how-to and I mean a LITERAL one. Don't feel bad. I wish I had one because it would have made my natural hair journey smoother.

Going natural is something new, and that can be quite scary. Yes, many of us were natural as little girls, but we weren't caring for our own hair and there were few products that actually nurtured our curls, coils and kinks. Times have changed. There are multitudes of support and tons of products out here to care for our natural texture.

So, how do you go natural? Here's a quick how-to that will ease your mind as you take the amazing leap and care for your natural tresses.

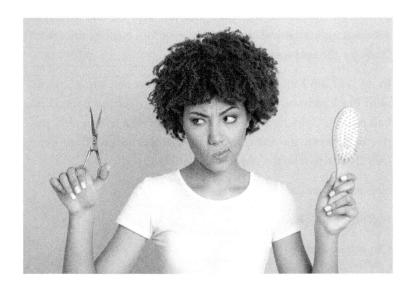

PICKING BETWEEN THE BIG CHOP OR LONG-TERM TRANSITIONING

Once you've made the choice to go natural, you have two options to choose from – The Big Chop or Transitioning. This needs to be the very first step in going natural with black hair. This step will determine what type of products you use, whether or not to cut your hair and how your journey will transpire. Let's find out what is expected from you for both paths. We will discuss each further in the next chapter.

Neither pathway is better. They are two options to going natural and you just need to decide which one is better for you and your lifestyle. Also, there is no time limit on how long to transition or when to BC. Choose for yourself and you can go as short as two months to as long as two years. So, just know, this is your journey and choice.

GET THE RIGHT TOOLS FOR NATURAL HAIR

Once you've decided on an approach to going natural, you must then equip yourself with the right styling tools and products. If I am being completely honest, the only thing that crossed over was a wide-tooth comb and my hooded dryer. If you just cannot bring yourself to trash it all, donate it to a women's shelter or simply give it away to friends and family members who may find a use for it. Now, no one is saying to break the bank with new products, but we do have a list of tools that most naturals use and need on day one.

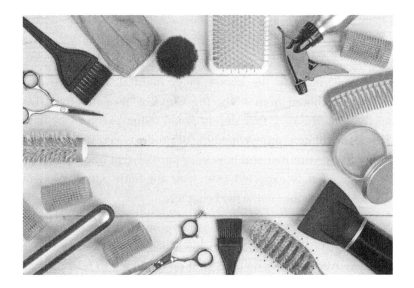

- Wide-tooth comb
- Moisturizing conditioner
- processing caps (cheap plastic caps)
- Satin sleeping bonnet and/or satin pillowcase
- Clarifying Shampoo
- Co-wash conditioner
- Deep conditioner
- Leave-in conditioner
- Styling gel and/or styling cream

Other products that some naturals find necessary are Magnetic rollers, Flexi rods, Denman brush or a tangle teezer. We delve deeper into the types of tools and why they might be required in chapter 4.

DITCH THE BAD STUFF!

While you begin buying new products, you must also get rid of all relaxers and chemical treatments from your home. If you decide to keep them, you may be tempted to use them. I do not use any of the hair products I used before going natural. I was caring for a very different type of hair and my relaxed hair had needs that are different from my natural tresses.

Sticking with the familiar or backsliding to relaxers is less likely if you ditch some products and tools that are not for natural hair. Here's a list of what to get rid of, since you will not have a need for them anymore.

- Relaxers - Obvious, but if you overlook removing this, you may be setting yourself up to backslide.
- Hair products specifically for relaxed hair - most of them do not address all the needs of natural hair.
- Rat tail comb - Maybe. Some still use them for parting their hair, but never and I mean NEVER comb your natural hair in its natural state with a rat tail comb. You will only be yanking out hair.
- Regular brushes - there are specific brushes for natural hair that are created to work with your natural tresses and not against them.
- Blow dryer **without** a diffuser - Either buy a diffuser or get a blow dryer with a diffuser attachment. A diffuser allows the heat from the dryer to speeds up drying time while maintaining your hair's natural curl pattern. They also keep heat from directly hitting your tresses.

CHANGE YOUR MINDSET ABOUT HAIR & HAIR CARE

You may think you have it all understood about going natural, but rocking relaxed hair for years has you with a relaxed hair mindset. Natural hair is the opposite of relaxed hair so you will need to rethink how to care for your hair. One of the biggest obstacles women find when going natural is how important moisture is to their hair and how water is the absolute BEST moisturizer around.

Good old-fashioned water is the best and simplest moisturizer on the planet. Natural hair needs water to maintain its elasticity or the ability to stretch. It nourishes our strands and many, if not the majority of products for our strands have water as the very first ingredient. This is just one step in understanding your natural hair and its needs. Our hair also needs protein. There is a delicate balance between moisture and protein that we delve further into in Chapter 6.

Be open to new ways of caring for your hair, and enlist a willingness to learn what your hair needs. Many women fail at going natural but often, it is due to their inability to understand the makeup of hair when it is in its natural state, and not being patient with their transition process. Let's discuss more next.

REMEMBER, THIS IS A JOURNEY. NOT A RACE!

One of the most important steps to going natural with your beautiful black hair is realizing that this is not a race but rather, a lifestyle change. Mastering going natural overnight is not realistic. I am STILL learning. I've been natural, going on 12 years! As we age, our hair needs change. Factor in hair changes due to hormonal, medical, and even geographical locals and seasons, and you can see why it will take a while for you to master natural hair.

Listen… you didn't master relaxed hair overnight. So please do not expect to do it with natural hair. Enlist patience, acceptance (of one's natural texture), and failures while you learn how to care for natural tresses. There are many wins when going natural but there is a lot of trial and error too. If you don't want to be one that goes natural several times, take your time, learn from your mistakes, and be patient with your hair and yourself.

If you want a positive outcome and healthy natural hair, then following these first steps will get you there. I love being natural and know you will too, so stay positive, open-minded and enjoy your natural hair journey once you choose to take the right steps to get you there!

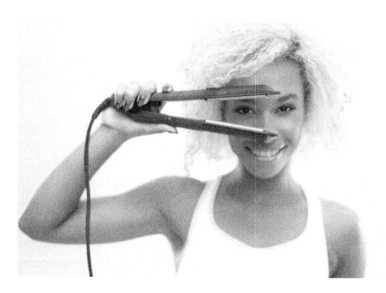

STEER CLEAR OF DIRECT HEAT FOR NATURAL HAIR

Your hair will be delicate while going from a relaxed to natural state. Your hair may seem like it's going through a transformation and many women incur dryness, breakage and shedding. This is the time to handle your hair with kid gloves. As you remove dangerous chemicals from your routine, adding heat can only cause more harm than good. Direct heat (flat irons, curling irons, straightening combs, blow dryers - without diffusers) dry out and damage curly, coily and kinky hair.

By now you have probably heard about heat damage and why you don't want it. An overly simplistic definition would be: Hair damage is "hair damaged by heat", but let's delve into what it is, what causes it and how to avoid it. Heat damage is hair that has had heat-styling tools set on temperatures too high, for too long, have been passed over too many times (or all of the above), and the hair has lost its natural elasticity.

This damages the hair shaft and changes its original curl, coil or kink. Heat damage is irreversible AND there is no such thing as heat training. If your hair does not revert back to it's natural coil, kink or coil, it has incurred heat damage. This can occur from one bad application of direct heat (flat iron, blow dryer without diffuser and pressing comb).

These tools, although convenient, are harsh on the hair and dry it out so the much-needed moisture our hair needs is depleted. We should be using direct heat sparingly (once a month or less) as even one application of direct heat can cause heat damage. If using direct heat, make sure to use a heat protectant and preferably one with silicones as silicones create a barrier to protect the hair from the heat-styling tool. Direct heat can be damaging to anyone's hair but when newly natural, your hair is weakened by chemicals (especially if transitioning and holding onto two very different textures).

No one is saying to leave heat alone forever, but give your hair a fighting chance as you go natural and care for it. Natural hair needs a ton of moisture. I mean a ton! Indirect heat like heating caps, blow dryers with diffusers, on low heat or cool, are the ideal ways of applying heat to your hair to stave off heat damage and dryness. You can also straighten your hair without heat (although it won't be bone straight), but we do have some tricks that will give you straight hair. Consider roller sets, and then you can wrap your hair like you used to do when relaxed.

CHAPTER THREE

SHOULD I BIG CHOP OR TRANSITION?

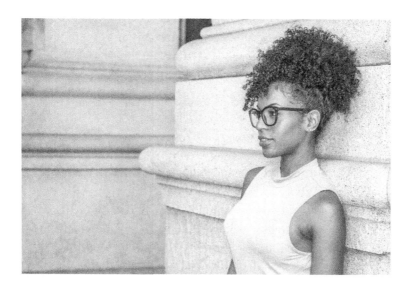

Going Natural is a wonderful journey to take. It's a personal one too, and each woman must determine how she will go about doing it. I grow weary of hearing far too many women say the journey is hard, long and full of pitfalls. Honestly, isn't life? I'm just feeling we need to be truthful about "Going Natural" and even if you are on round 2, 3 or even 4, understand very few things in life that are worth it, take little to no effort.

One of the first choices to make going natural is the path you choose. There are two main routes to take, and neither is better than the other. I am going to give you in-depth information on both.

THE BIG CHOP

The Big Chop is cutting off all relaxed hair or chemically treated strands. Understandably, this may be a daunting prospect if you have never worn your hair cropped before, but many ladies have described the experience as freeing. So if you are brave and impulsive, this is the path for you. Doing the Big Chop (BC) can be done by you or a professional, especially if you are looking for a specific style to rock while starting out the gate.

WOMEN WHO ARE INTERESTED IN THE BIG CHOP

- Not wanting to deal with their relaxed ends. If you are over your relaxed hair and just want to ditch it, then the BC is for you!
- Women who do not want to take care of two different textures nor do they want to find styles that help both textures look uniform.
- Women who love short hair. Hey, there are all kinds and if you love short hair, cut it off and have fun with the tons of accessories around to do it up anyway you see fit, and that includes added hair.
- You have severely damaged hair. This may be the best route for you. Start with a clean slate by doing the BC and know that you can bring your hair back to being healthy.

HOW TO DO THE BIG CHOP?

There are a couple of ways to tackle this task. First off, don't do like me and just start cutting when angry at your damaged hair. That's a serious no, no. Instead, take a smart approach. You can do it yourself or enlist the help of a professional hairstylist.

If you choose to do it yourself (DIY):

- Start on freshly washed hair. It is easier to see both relaxed and natural textures and makes for an easier cut.
- Section hair into 4 or more sections to make sure all permed ends get cut and allows for easier manipulation of the hair.
- Use hair shears, not just any scissors laying around, so you can get even and unfrayed ends.
- Simply cut the permed ends off section by section.

Now, hopefully your hair is even or at least in a place to rock a style like a TWA. If not or if you are in need of a style, head over to a professional natural hair stylist.

If you choose to go to a hairstylist for your BC, simply book a consultation with a stylist who is knowledgeable in cutting natural hair. Have them remove all the permed ends and get a style. Either way is workable.

LONG-TERM TRANSITIONING OR TRANSITIONING

The object is to keep your hair length while going natural. There are no hard and fast rules on how long to transition, so go as long as you feel comfortable with the transition. You decide on how long to transition, though many go for at least one year while some wait even longer. There is no perfect time to transition, so do not feel locked into a set length of time.

Some women considering going natural feel transitioning is harder as you are working with two textures. Well actually, three when you factor in scab hair. Scab hair is the unscientific term associated with the newly grown hair that comes in after one stops using relaxers. It's very fragile, dry and prone to breakage but may not even remotely resemble your natural tresses. Now, BC'ing will not keep you from dealing with the scab hair but you don't have to worry about the relaxed ends along with it.

WOMEN WHO ARE INTERESTED IN TRANSITIONING

- Women not ready to cut all of their hair off. It's not for everyone and going natural has to feel comfortable for you. If keeping your tresses is going to make that transition easier, then by all means do it!
- Women who hate short hair or hate it on them. It takes some of us longer to get those longer tresses, so don't feel like you have to sport a TWA for anyone.
- The woman whose significant other (SO) needs time for adjustment. Or maybe you need the time to adjust. There are several women who complain their SO doesn't want them to go natural. Well, you can slowly go into it and give all parties involved a chance to see just how beautiful this journey is.
- The woman who wants to practice on styles. Yes, there will be more styles to work with as a Long-Term Transitioner since you will have more hair to work with. Curlier styles work best when long-term transitioning as it's easier to blend relaxed, scab, and natural hair on curlier styles than straight styles.

HOW TO TRANSITION?

If you choose to transition and not BC, you are giving the go ahead to either snip your permed ends slowly (some will snip ½ inch to an inch of hair monthly) or wait. You can pick when to chop all the remaining permed ends at once yourself. (some choose to wait at least six months to one year but there are some waiting even longer like two years.)

There is no right or wrong length of time. Whether you wait two months or two years, transition for as long as you feel comfortable. Remember...this is YOUR journey. No one else can take it for you, so let's keep it as positive and pleasant as possible. Both routes are great but may be filled with setbacks or pitfalls. Reason being, this is something new to you AND your hair. Patience, love, gentleness and knowledge is necessary for you to succeed, so first things first...pick your route and look forward to a beautiful transformation!

CHAPTER FOUR

HAIR PRODUCTS & TOOLS INCLUDING POPULAR NATURAL OILS

This may be the most expensive endeavor for a new natural outside of styling especially when first taking the plunge. For this reason, I would not go natural when broke, but don't feel you have to be flush either. Just make sure you can pick up a few things to make your journey easier. Here's a list of what most naturals need when first starting out, followed by a description of each item:

- Cleansers - Co-wash, Sulfate-free, clarifying
- Conditioners - Rinse out (regular), deep, leave-in
- Stylers
- Processing Caps
- Satin Bonnet and/or Satin pillowcase
- Spray Bottle
- Microfiber towel
- Wide-tooth comb

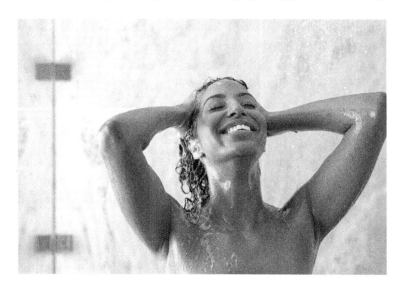

CO-WASHING CONDITIONER (CO-WASH)

Many new naturals are confused on the whole co-wash/shampoo debate, but I am here to explain why both products, a co-wash and a shampoo, are still necessary when going natural. First off, the co-washing conditioner or co-wash is a staple product for most naturals.

A co-wash is for washing the hair with a cleansing conditioner or a botanical conditioner. In recent years, beauty companies have begun creating products labeled "co-wash" that are designed to clean and condition the hair. These commercial co-wash products may contain cleansing agents (surfactants), but are usually less harsher than those found in shampoo. Shampoo is necessary to clean hair but quite often uses harsh surfactants that strips the natural oils from curly or kinky hair, and our strands NEED those natural oils. A cleansing conditioner or co-wash does the job using natural ingredients and with cleanser that are less harsh. That is why many of them have no suds or low suds.

A co-wash is the foundation of the Curly Girl Method, which is a unique way to care for curly/coily/kinky hair. I've used it, loved it because it provided a hybrid of the method with huge success. This does not mean I never use shampoo, however. Some instances require the use of a deeper cleanings product.

SULFATE-FREE SHAMPOO

A sulfate-free shampoo is free of sulfates or primary surfactants, but does cleanse the hair. Sulfate-free shampoos are just milder detergents that don't completely wash away hair's much needed moisture. Most do not lather (but still clean) and are great for 3 & 4 hair textures or color-treated hair.

Some naturals prefer just using a sulfate-free shampoo to get the benefits of a cleanser without the harshness of a regular shampoo. They are great for anyone who just doesn't subscribe to using a co-wash or likes to switch between the two from time to time.

CLARIFYING SHAMPOO

A clarifying shampoo is an ultra-cleansing shampoo that removes all traces of dirt and product build-up, while is also needed for removing hard water deposits and chlorine. This is the type of shampoo you need to use after going swimming. They are relatively new to many black women, but so are a lot of products that we didn't even realize we needed before, just like heat protectant. Clarifying shampoos are just deep cleaning shampoos that work extra hard to rid hair of all the bad stuff.

They are necessary because they rid hair of all the extra gunk, dirt, pollutants, metals and chlorine that comes in contact with our hair. They may not be needed for every wash but when hair needs that extra cleaning, it's time to pull out the big guns. They are especially necessary if you have hard water or go swimming in the ocean or a pool.

I use a clarifying shampoo when swimming or when I have neglected to wash my hair for a long time (*gasp) or used silicones that just sit on my hair and need them removed. Some women simply prefer shampoos because they don't feel that co-washing gets their hair clean enough and while that is perfectly fine, you may want to stick with sulfate-free shampoos to prevent dryness and scalp irritation.

I have and use both. I use co-wash conditioners for regular washdays and use a clarifying shampoo when swimming or hair is ultra-dirty. Never feel you have to only use one but instead, listen to what your hair needs. You will hear me say that A LOT! Your hair is the biggest guide on what you need so pay attention to it, and you will be just fine.

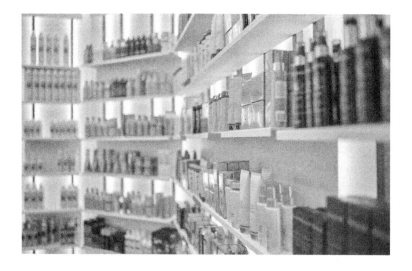

MOISTURIZING CONDITIONER OR RINSE-OUT CONDITIONER

Moisturizing conditioners are just regular or rinse-out conditioners we have been using for years! Every curly girl needs to use a rinse out conditioner because it keeps our hair moisturized in the days after styling. The natural oils from our scalp don't travel all the way down our hair shaft because of our curl pattern. This creates dryness. So we coat our hair with a rinse out conditioner so that it will stay moisturized in order for us to retain length.

If you're complaining of dry hair and you don't use a rinse out conditioner – here's why. The conditioner closes our hair cuticle and keeps the moisture locked in after the shampoo has lifted and stripped our cuticles. The closed cuticle makes it less susceptible to breakage when detangling with your fingers or combs. The conditioner makes our hair easy to detangle because of the 'slip' that comes with this heavy product, since the rinse out conditioner is heavier than a leave-in.

Our hair will stay moisturized, even though we rinse it out; therefore: leaving it in our hair is not good, unless it is a botanical conditioner. The label should tell you whether to rinse it out, keep it in or if you can do either and yes, there are some that you can do both.

DEEP CONDITIONER

Deep conditioners are penetrating conditioners that add moisture, maintains elasticity, and strengthens the hair strands on a deeper level. They actually penetrate the hair shaft. Not all products have this ability. That's the magic behind a deep conditioner and the reason they are necessary on every single washday. They are there to not only protect and keep hair moisturized but also combat the damages you inflict on your hair during washing, styling and regular day-to-day wear.

A regular conditioner or rinse-out is not a deep conditioner because it won't penetrate the hair shaft and affect hair on a deeper level. Deep conditioners have fortifying ingredients that should be free from drying alcohol, parabens, and mineral oil. It should have humectants and emollients such as oils and good fatty alcohols such as cetearyl alcohol. Regular conditioners are not created to work as hard as their counterparts so you will not be getting the benefits by using that alone.

I cannot tell you how often I have to tell new naturals (and not so new) that they need to be using a deep conditioner on EVERY SINGLE WASH DAY! This product is critical to maintain strong and healthy hair.

LEAVE-IN CONDITIONER

Leave-in's are light, water-based conditioners that have been specially formulated to allow for more frequent use than regular rinse-out conditioners. Rinse-out and deep conditioners contain ingredients that are designed to bind to the hair after rinsing. This can lead to product build-up if regular conditioners are used often and without rinsing.

Leave-in conditioners don't require rinsing and can be used daily without excessive build-up. Many leave-in conditioners contain humectants, which draw water into the hair. This makes these types of conditioners perfect for moisturizing and preventing dryness. Basically, using a leave-in protects and hydrates your hair for lasting moisture and style.

A quick tip is mixing some leave-in conditioner, water and an essential or carrier oil in a water bottle, mostly water. Use the mixture as a refresher in the morning or at night when twisting or braiding hair.

STYLER

We all have to style our hair and learn what products you need to give our hair the hold or look we want. Now, do not confuse this with creating curls. There is no product on the market that can create curls. There are products that will enhance, tighten or loosen them. There are also styles that will give you curls like rod sets, roller sets, braid and twist outs. I will discuss them in a later chapter.

Stylers provide shape and hold by adding a film on the hair that creates natural bonds between neighboring strands while holding them in place. Stylers give your style hold, de-frizz and enhance your definition. There are a few that most naturals gravitate to for this big job because most of us want our style to last and we need the moisture to stay in. These products help.

- *Curl (Defining) Cream* - puddings, custards, soufflés, and all other opaque stylers are great for capturing your natural coil and for setting your wash-and-gos, twists or braid outs. They may have a light, medium or heavy hold and the package will guide you. Many Type 3s use these types of stylers.
- *Mousse or Foam* - are in the same family as setting and styling lotions. Many of us used them for roller sets while relaxed and you can use them again for those same styles while natural. These products offer more touchable results and are much lighter than gels or pomades.
- *Styling Gel* - my go-to for wash-and-gos, styling gels, is not the same gels from yesteryear. They are lighter, not sticky and no longer have the drying effects of alcohol that made them flaky and hard. Styling gels create a stronger hold than styling creams and are great for Type 4 hair. Many of today's gels use sliptastic ingredients like aloe vera gel, flaxseed gel, marshmallow root, and slippery elm to hold hair while allowing it to stay soft and shiny.
- *Heat Protectant* - Something new to many naturals, heat protectants, adds moisture to hair while forming a

protective barrier to your strands when heat is applied. Yes, we should have been using this years ago, but only recently have we even realized the need for it because we do not want heat damage! **Heat damage** is irreversible damage to the strand. If your hair does not revert back to it's natural coil, kink or curl, it has incurred heat damage. Cutting it off is the only remedy for this problem, so use the lowest setting possible. Use heat protectant and pass through the hair once if using a flat iron. *Always, and I mean ALWAYS apply heat protectant before using any direct heat to your hair.*

- *Pomade or Butter* - Another product for those twists and braid outs, known as pomade and butter, are heavier stylers ideal for Type 4 hair. They are loaded with butters and oils to help seal in moisture while holding your style in place and even adding sheen.

- *Edge Tamer* - While every edge tamer is NOT created equal, the product is designed to lay down those edges for a smooth and sleek look. Natural hair is not as controllable as relaxed hair so many women struggle with the right edge tamer and how to allow those edges to lay. The right edge tamer (along with a trick of tying a silk scarf or bandana around the edges for a few minutes or hours) lends naturals to laid edges and/or baby hair that many have loved while relaxed.

This is a better choice than relaxing your edges for the same effect as relaxing your edges only defeats the purpose of going natural and will only lend to damaging your hair. This product is completely optional and I have only started using an edge tamer within the last year or so, and I've been natural for over eleven years.

PROCESSING CAPS (CHEAP PLASTIC CAPS)

Many of us already have these caps around for deep condition-ings, and typically use as shower caps or for dying hair. They are cheaper than cheap, so make sure to keep them around because they are GREAT for deep conditioning sessions, hot oil treat-ments or a pre poo session. A pre poo is an oil treatment prior to washing your hair to help with detangling or to combat the negative effects of shampooing hair. Processing caps are always good, so keep them around.

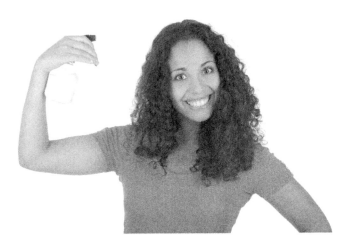

SPRAY BOTTLE

We all need a spray bottle and I JUST got on my sister the other day for not having one! I have several and each serves a specific purpose. A natural needs moisture and the best moisturizer in the world is water. A spray bottle is excellent for refreshing your hair in the morning when you fluff or need to fully rewet your hair (without getting in the shower) or at night to help braid or twist up your hair for the next day. The spray bottle evenly mists your hair without having to fully rewet it. I have one with just water and lavender oil; I double it as a face refresher in the morning too. I also have one with a leave-in conditioner, glycerin and lavender oil mix for a DIY refresher when I need a light misting to keep my hair from frizzing.

You don't need anything fancy and can pick one up from any beauty supply place; however, they do have hair misters for this kind of thing if you just want one. The bottom line is every natural will eventually need or use one of those things, and you will surely see a difference when you keep them around.

SATIN SLEEPING BONNET AND/OR SATIN PILLOWCASE

I'm sure you've seen the memes of a black woman with her satin bonnet on her head proclaiming she's in for the night. In many instances, a satin bonnet has become synonymous with natural hair. Protecting natural hair is priority. That means sleeping on satin or silk is imperative. Cotton sheets or pillowcases create friction and dry out hair. They can also mess up hairstyles; therefore, wearing a satin bonnet, scarf or using a satin pillowcase is required to protect hair while sleeping.

They can be found at any BSS, Beauty Supply Store, but with the surge of women going natural, there has been a surge in the entrepreneurial spirit. Many black women have created satin bonnets and scarves just for us. I take this step very seriously and have a satin scarf and sleep on a satin pillowcase. Investing in satin-lined hats and beanies is also a great idea as wool or cotton hats will have the same disastrous effects.

MICROFIBER HAIR-DRYING TOWEL OR OLD T-SHIRT

Just as cotton sheets and pillowcases are detrimental to natural hair, regular bath towels are just as damaging. On washday, we often dry our hair with whatever towel we can find when relaxed but with natural hair, those same bath towels cause friction, frizz and breakage to natural tresses. Microfiber hair towels are designed for natural hair, to not disturb the curl or create friction. There are lot of brands out here to aid in hair drying, which range in prices.

If you just do not want to spend money, an old t-shirt has a smoother texture and will prevent frizz. I used one for years until I found the right towel for me. Before jumping into this investment, use an old t-shirt until you find the right hair drying towel for you.

WIDE-TOOTH COMB

A wide tooth comb is exactly what it sounds like - a comb with wide spaces between the teeth. The teeth are not necessarily bigger (although some combs do come that way) but the wider spaces allow our kinkier texture to be detangled or combed with less friction. That means less hairs in your comb and more on your head! A wide-tooth comb helps prevent/reduce frayed ends, makes it easier to detangle and creates less frizz. This is a necessary tool when going natural, whether transitioning or doing the BC.

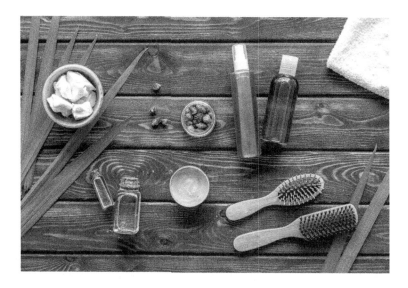

POPULAR NATURAL OILS

Natural oils are loved and used often by naturals. With the boom in recent years, you are likely to find women with straight and relaxed hair jumping on our bandwagon. Naturals love and use both essential oils (a natural oil typically obtained by distillation from a plant or herb, and often very potent) and carrier oils (vegetable oil derived from the fatty portion of a plant and often used to dilute the potency of essential oils). Here are some of the most popular and beneficial to natural hair.

Amla Oil - Amla has medicinal and anti-cariogenic properties. A natural powerhouse of goodness, Alma is rich in Vitamin C, Calcium, Phosphorus, Iron, Carotene, Vitamin B Complex and also a powerful antioxidant agent. This oil is excellent for fighting dandruff, increasing hair growth and conditioning.

Argan Oil - Argan oil is derived from the argan tree nuts from the native Argan tree in Morocco. Known as "liquid gold", this oil has been used as a skin moisturizer and hair conditioner since ancient times. Argan oil has a unique composition with an more than 200% tocopherols (Vitamin E) than olive oil and has very high levels of fatty acids. Argan oil has Squalene, Polyphenols and Sterols. Argan oil is ideal for preventing dryness, adding sheen to strands, taming frizz and use during scalp massages.

Avocado Oil - Rich in potassium, Vitamin E, protein, Vitamin A, Vitamin K, fiber, folate, Vitamin B6, Vitamin C and protein, Avocado oil is a natural hair and skin healer. Since it is close to the natural composition of the oils our skin naturally produces, it is easily absorbs and is able to aid the skin and hair in healing. This is great when dealing with rough, cracked skin.

The fatty richness of avocado is good for healing, moisturizing, and protecting the hair as it contains most of the nutrients and vitamins that are produced in our sebum. Because of this fact, the oil is absorbed easily into the hair and scalp so that it seals in moisture and protects the hair from the elements.

Castor Oil (Jamaican Black Castor Oil) - Obtained from the castor bean, Castor oil is an ideal solution for better hair growth. This 100% pure, natural and unadulterated oil is packed with various vital elements such as vitamin E, minerals, proteins, anti-fungal properties and more. Castor oil has been proven helpful for controlling hair loss, fighting scalp infections and combating dandruff.

Coconut Oil - Coconut oil is extracted oil from the fruit (coconut) of the coconut tree. An edible oil, it has been consumed in tropical places for thousands of years. It benefits our bodies from inside out and despite what most know about this oil, there is more than just one type.

- **Unrefined (virgin) coconut oil** – retains the original coconut's chemical composition. It's made from fresh coconut meat and considered superior to the other two forms.
- **Refined coconut oil** – is made from dried coconut meat

that has been bleached, deodorized, treated and processed through high temperatures extract flavor and aroma. While some nutrients are stripped, the fatty acid composition is untouched.

- **Fractionated coconut oil** – most are unaware of this type that stays in liquid form and is only a fraction of coconut oil. Just about all of the long chain triglycerides are removed through hydrolysis and steam distillation.

Coconut oil is rich in carbohydrates, vitamins and minerals. For a long time, it was demonized by it's high saturated fat content. People are beginning to think differently about this oil as those saturated fats are handled differently in our bodies. It has healthy fats or good fats called medium-chain fatty acids (MCFAs) like Caprylic acid, Lauric acid and Capric acid. The bottom-line: Populations that eat a lot of coconut oil are healthier.

Jojoba Oil - The highly enchanting Jojoba oil, obtained from the jojoba plant, is considered to be a wonderful choice as its constituents slightly resembles sebum that is naturally produced by our scalps. This means that, most likely, your scalp will readily accept jojoba oil without showing any side effects. The soothing and moisturizing effects of this oil treats the hair follicles from deep inside, which is proven helpful in keeping your hair dandruff free.

Lavender Oil - Lavender oil is stimulating, meaning that it increases circulation to the scalp. Not only does that encourage new hair growth, but it also provides much needed nutrients and oxygen to the root of the hair, which makes the root stronger and reduces the amount of shedding. This oil also combats against nits and lice, which can also lead to hair falling out. Much like its counterparts, it also contains antibacterial properties that wards off infections, fungi and unwanted bacteria.

Olive Oil - Olive oil has been used for centuries as a tool for beautiful hair, skin and nails. Packed full of Vitamin E and A, olive oil has amazing anti-aging properties. Olive oil treats inflammation and acne, and also aids in the moisturizing excessively dry skin and hair. This oil has the power to both regenerate skin cells and help improve the elasticity of the skin. The best way to reap the full benefits of its anti-aging properties is to apply a small amount of olive oil to your skin before heading to bed on a daily basis.

In addition to that, olive oil also promotes hair growth, acts as a natural conditioner, imparts shine and treats itchy scalp and dandruff. The latter is especially important to keep in mind during the winter months. Due to its thick nature, olive oil is a great component to add to your hair care regimen if you're looking to protect your hair from harsh, colder climates.

Sweet Almond Oil - Almond oil is known to be a natural "moisturizer" due to its softening properties. Sweet Almond oil contains Vitamins E and D, along with a host of other minerals including calcium and magnesium. This makes almond oil one of the only oils that can prevent the hair from drying out and becoming brittle. Dry, brittle hair has a tendency to break and fall out very easily. Incorporating almond oil into your regimen will not only provide your hair with some much needed nutrition, but it will also ensure that the hair stays strong and grows in faster.

CHAPTER FIVE

HOW TO WASH NATURAL HAIR

Clean hair is the best pathway to healthy hair. Please take heed to the old myth that dirty hair grows faster has been debunked. We really need to just leave that way of thinking in the past! We use a lot of products in our hair; not to mention, just everyday pollutants and dirt that all need to be removed from our strands. Washing natural hair is a big deal and while we are all experts at washing relaxed hair, natural is different and you need to know how to properly cleanse natural or transitioning strands.

Natural hair does not fall, act or even look like relaxed hair so we should not expect to wash it in the same fashion. While there are a few variations on how to actually wash natural hair, we will be discussing the most basic and most used methods.

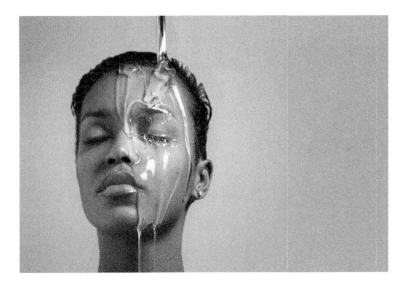

Prep with a Pre-Poo - Prior to even washing your hair, you must protect it from the harshness of cleansing our hair. Shampoo with it's surfactants can be very drying and damaging to our delicate strands. Shampoos are designed to clean the hair by ridding it of all oil, dirt and build-up. In order to do this, many commercial shampoos contain detergents and cleaning agents, such as sodium laureth sulfate. This is why many naturals choose to wash with cleansing conditioners.

Another way to combat those effects is to simply do a pre-poo. Pre-pooing before washing makes hair easier to detangle, but it also keeps hair moisturized after it's been shampooed. The best pre-poos are usually natural ingredients like oils, creams and some fruits that are beneficial to hair health, such as avocado. Pre-pooing is very helpful if you constantly have to battle with your hair while detangling, due to a dry or brittle texture.

HOW TO DO A PRE-POO

I often get this question, as many women appreciate a step by step explanation.

1. Section hair into at least four sections. Take your time if hair is tangled as you do not want to rip any strands out. You can lightly spray hair to help.
2. If hair is very thick, you can split each section into twos and then start applying your pre-poo by starting at the ends and working your way up the hair shaft. Apply the oil liberally, and your tangles should be removed as you add the pre-poo.
3. This is a prime time to detangle your hair after you've applied the pre-poo thoroughly to your sectioned hair. You can use your fingers, a tangle tool or brush.
4. Once detangled, you can go onto the next section by following the same steps. If you plan on keeping hair in the pre-poo overnight, place each detangled section in twists to keep from detangling.
5. To make the pre-poo more effective, cover with a plastic cap and add heat. You could also consider using a thermal cap or sitting under a hooded dryer for at least 15 minutes, though you can keep it in longer. Once you are ready, wash your hair and your hair should be well moisturized and detangled.

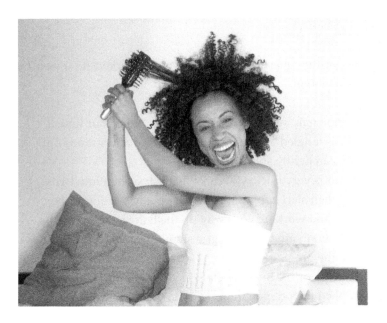

Detangling (removing tangles) - Detangling is a chore for many naturals yet for others, it is like a four letter word! Natural hair is coily, curly and kinky. Those hairs coil around other strands, and itself, to create tangles for days. This is the reason some naturals opt for stretched or straight styles to decrease the tangles. When it comes to washdays, however, all bets are off. You must deal with detangling to have a productive washday and style.

Some women prefer detangling prior to cleansing hair, and enlist the assistance of a pre-poo, but there are others who prefer to do it when they are conditioning their hair.

Which way is more effective?

The path that works for you. Trial and error will almost always be your guide.

Pre-Wash Detangling

Detangling the hair before shampooing is a great method to use if you've just taken your hair out of twists or braids.

Removing the bulk of the shedded hair beforehand will reduce the amount of breakage and tangling you might experience if you waited to detangle your hair later on in the washing process.

This method is also great if you prefer to wash your hair while it's plaited, due to the fact that it ensures the amount of tangles formed will be significantly less than usual. Some naturals prefer this method when they have put off washday a tad too long and know some of those tangles need to be worked on prior to shampooing, which can create tangles on its own.

Post-Wash Detangling

If you ask any number of naturals, most opt to detangle the hair after it has been shampooed and doused in the conditioner of their choice. Whether it's with a wide toothed comb or your fingers, the best part about this method is the fact that the conditioner provides slippage and makes the hair softer, making it easier to detangle the hair. Detangling post-shampoo will also guarantee that you won't have to detangle twice, but it will leave a lot of shedded hair in the drain.

There are tools specifically created for detangling that include combs, brushes and even products. Ask ten naturals what they use to detangle and you will very likely get ten different tools or techniques. Just like washing hair, work in sections and try not to get aggravated with your tangles. Improper detangling (going to fast, yanking, working on dry hair) will yield in you removing more than shedded hair and tangles.

Tips to detangling properly:

Take your time. This is not a race so make sure to detangle when you have the energy, time and are in the right mood. You can watch a movie, listen to music or just do whatever you like to pass the time while detangling.

Allow your oils, conditioner or water to help! They help the process go smoothly and as a benefit, will help you lose less healthy hair.

No yanking or pulling. Just don't do it. You will end up pulling more than your shedded hair.

No dry detangling. Your hair needs something to make it smoother and allow the tangles to loosen up. Use products with great slip or glide through the hair easily to make for an effective detangling session. Do not detangle your dry hair!

Use a sulfate-free shampoo, co-wash or clarifying shampoo - I want to explain that at one time or another you will use all of those types of cleansers for your natural hair, depending on what your hair needs at the moment. On regular wash days, I use a co-wash. On days when my hair needs extra cleanings, I use a sulfate-free shampoo. On days I need to detoxify my hair or remove hard water or chlorine, I use a clarifying shampoo. Your hair will determine which type to use.

Wash hair in sections - Unless you are rocking a really short TWA, this is a must for a more pleasant washday experience! Our hair knots up. Washing in sections can alleviate some of our hair trauma by working with it instead of working against it. This will also keep us from spending too much time on washing. Once the hair is long enough (about 6 inches in length), you will find this technique helpful.

Section the hair into at least four parts with a wide-tooth comb or your fingers, but it can be sectioned into 6 or even 8 if need be. This may be necessary for our thicker-hair Naturals. Braid each section to keep them separate or ban them if braiding is not your thing. Wash each braid separately. You can leave it braided or unbraided when working on each section, but make sure to re-braid or re-band when moving onto the next section. Rinse each section separately. You can apply conditioner in the same manner as the shampoo. I usually keep sections until I apply leave-in. By then, hair is tangle-free and willing to play nice. Now it is time to head over to the conditioning part of the wash day!

Using LOC or LCO on washday - LOC (Liquid + Oil + Cream) or LCO (Liquid + Cream + Oil) - applications are to retain moisture in natural hair. Both methods are highly effective at keeping natural strands moisturized by applying the liquid and then the cream and oil in either fashion. This is pivotal to long-lasting moisturized hair until your next washday. i

THE STEP BY STEP GUIDE FOR WASHDAY

Many new naturals prefer a guide on when and how to wash natural hair, so I put together an outline to help. Now, wash days vary though for most naturals, this step by step guide is how your washday will go.

1. Hair should be washed regularly and for most, that is twice a month. Washing hair weekly may be too often for many naturals as too much washing can dry out your hair's moisture. If hair is dirty or coated with products before your usual washday, then wash your hair and make sure to do a pre-poo to keep hair moisturized. You can also alternate between a shampoo and a co-wash, if you want to wash weekly or more.
2. On wash day, have your tools ready. Pre-poo, shampoo (or co-wash), deep conditioner, leave-in conditioner and styling products. A wide tooth comb, detangling tool, cheap plastic cap, thermal cap or hooded dryer, microfiber towel and hair clips are also necessary.
3. Pick a day you have time for the entire process as for many, wash day can take hours from start to finish with detangling and drying being the most time spent. Many

naturals will cut the time down by doing a pre-poo or
the deep conditioning overnight.

4. Start with the pre-poo. Instructions can be found in an
   earlier section of the chapter. Detangle well while hair is
   in the pre-poo.
5. Next, you can either wash your hair in the shower or in
   the kitchen sink.
6. Saturate your hair well for 2-3 minutes prior to washing
   as the long rinse will loosen up product build-up, dirt
   and even some remaining tangles.
7. Hair should already be sectioned from the pre-poo stage
   so take each section down and begin applying a quarter
   to silver dollar size of cleansers to your scalp and
   massage with your finger tips. Never use your nails!
   Allow the cleanser to run down the rest of your hair or
   simply run it down the length of your hair to ensure all
   product and dirt is removed. Massage your scalp well
   moving in a downward motion and not in circles as that
   can encourage tangles. Once the section is fully cleansed,
   twist up that section and move onto the next section.
8. Continue until all sections are clean and then return to
   the first section you washed to take down and rinse.
   Rinse in sections to discourage tangles. Rinse well to
   ensure all cleanser is removed and then you can twist it
   up again and repeat the steps. Take your time rinsing
   hair to ensure all cleaner is gone.
9. Time to do some detangling with a detangler or rinse out
   conditioner. I suggest a cheap or less expensive one so
   you can use a lot to help with the detangling process.
   This is one of the longest steps for some naturals as some
   of us have more tangles than other. Pre-detangling prior
   to washing with a pre-poo helps to lessen this step so if
   you suffer from a lot of tangles, make the pre-poo a
   consistent part of wash day. Make sure to remove ALL
   tangles prior to moving onto the next step.

10. Time to deep condition. Apply a liberal amount to each section of hair (about a silver dollar or more) and start from the roots to the ends. Make sure all strands are covered. This is where you lather it on! You can finger-detangle once hair is coated or use a wide tooth comb to ensure all hairs are tangle free and full of DC. Place hair back in twist or out, and continue the same steps on the other sections of hair.

11. Once hair is completely covered, place the cheap plastic cap on your head and finish your shower (if in the shower). Now it is time to DC with heat! Use your thermal heat cap or a hooded dryer for at least 15 to 30 minutes to allow the DC to penetrate the hair shaft.

12. Time to rinse out the DC. Remove the cap and rinse out one section of hair at a time. Hair should be fully detangled and softer. By this point, you have prepped your hair for styling. Hair should be saturated or damp before adding your leave-in conditioner. You may rake it in, smooth it in or simply apply and comb it through.

13. The next steps vary as to the type of stylers and tools you chose, depending on the style you will be creating. That can be from a simple wash and go, to a flexi rod set to a straight style.

Wash day can be lengthy if you have thicker or longer hair, or even if you hair tends to tangle easily. Your style can also increase the time, especially styles like roller sets or twists. Whether it is short or long, make sure to fully detangle your hair and do a great job because a great washday yields amazing styles that last longer and look better. Keeping hair clean is important. Dirty hair does not grow faster and can actually create problems for your scalp and hair. Styles look better on clean hair, and it grows in a clean and healthy environment.

CHAPTER SIX

HOW TO CONDITION NATURAL HAIR

Conditioner is a huge component of the washday, and excellent for keeping our hair frizz-free, soft, manageable and healthy. Knowing what types of conditioners are needed for natural hair is just as important as knowing how to properly use them. It's not always about brand but also ingredient and intent.

Knowing the difference between a regular (rinse out), leave-in or deep conditioner is crucial to keeping your hair properly conditioned, moisturized and healthy overall. Here is a breakdown of the three conditioners, when to use them and how.

Every curly girl needs to use a **rinse out conditioner** because it keeps the hair moisturized in the days after styling. The natural oils from our scalp don't travel all the way down our hair shaft because of our curl pattern. We must coat our hair with a rinse out conditioner so that it will stay moisturized, in order for us to retain length.

If you're complaining of dry hair and you don't use a rinse out conditioner – here's why. The conditioner closes our hair cuticle and keeps the moisture locked in after the shampoo has lifted and stripped our cuticles. The closed cuticle makes it less susceptible to breakage when detangling with your fingers or comb. As well as, the conditioner makes our hair easy to detangle because of the 'slip' that comes with this heavy product as the rinse out conditioner is heavier than a leave-in. Our hair will stay moisturized, even though we rinse it out; therefore, leaving it in our hair is not good.

We should use a rinse out conditioner weekly to replace moisture lost throughout the week from the elements of the environment and our manipulation. If you want a moisturizing product to stay in your hair after wash day, use a leave in.

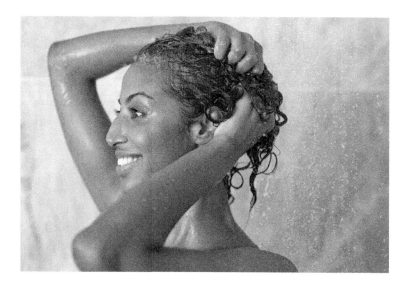

HOW TO USE A RINSE-OUT CONDITIONER

You mostly use a rinse out conditioner on washday. It not only assists in protecting your hair, but it is a great tool to use for detangling. Liberally apply the rinse out conditioner to sectioned hair, and either finger detangle or use a detangling tool like a wide-tooth comb to not only remove knots but to also fully distribute the product to all strands. You can also use them in between washes to refresh and re-moisturize hair. It's best to use a botanical conditioner as they will help your hair and scalp, and not weight down your strands. If your hair needs a real pick me up but not a real washing, opt for rewetting your hair, using a rinse-out conditioner and following up on your regular styling routine. This is a great option when you want to rock a wash-an-go or revive your twist-out.

If you want great moisture retention and elasticity – deep condition your hair every week with heat. The heat from a hooded dryer or a thermal cap causes the cuticles to be raised, and allows the emollients and moisturizing ingredients to fully penetrate and coat the hair shaft.

Everyone should **deep condition** their hair because it adds an extra boost of moisture and protection for the days after styling. It should be done every week but can be stretched to bi-weekly, depending on your hair preference. I suggest deep conditioning every single solitary wash day! You want to know why? Because of the hundreds of questions I get from readers who complain about their hair being brittle, dry or breaking off. They always and I mean always have neglected to make deep conditioning a part of their washday routine!

Deep conditioning fills the holes in the hair cuticle (which is a cause of poor porosity) from the damage and manipulation that occurred in the week and the parts that the regular conditioner may have missed. Deep conditioning on a regular basis adds shine, prevents dryness and damage, and improves the overall look, feel and health of your natural hair. I also suggest doing a deep conditioner with heat like a heat cap, a warm towel or a hooded dryer for 15 to 30 minutes. Yes, it may be a pain to put that much effort into the process, but the heat helps the conditioner to penetrate the hair shaft and impart all the moisturizing and strengthening ingredients from the DC into your hair. This is a huge benefit to keep hair stronger and healthier.

Last but certainly not least, we must discuss the leave-in conditioner. So, why do we use a **leave-in conditioner** if we use a rinse out conditioner and deep conditioner? Because the leave-in serves a real purpose. This lightweight product acts as a protective barrier around our hair shaft for when it is being manipulated during the styling process, affected due to the environmental conditions and rubbed against our cotton clothes.

In addition, it adds a bit of moisture for the days after styling. Ladies, please don't even consider just using leave-in conditioners (instead of the rinse out) because it simply isn't moisturizing enough as they have a higher water content and are lighter than a rinse out. They also will not work longer than a day or so. They can be used daily because they are lighter and make for better daily styling. A leave-in conditioner will bring your hair back to life from day to day and allow for easier styling. It will keep hair looking and feeling its best between washings.

Not quite a conditioner, but just as important in the washday process is the **protein treatment, masque or conditioner.** This is needed from time to time. Our hair is made up of a very hard protein called Keratin. We chip away at that protein by our day to day styling, including with heat. We also damage it when we color or use chemical straighteners. You rebuild that damaged protein by using protein treatments but not weekly or even monthly for many of us.

The more damage you inflict on your hair requires more usage of a protein treatment, though too much protein can cause hair to become brittle and break. I usually do a protein treatment every 2 to 3 months, since I never use heat-styling and steer clear of chemicals. For most folks, monthly is adequate.

CHAPTER SEVEN

HOW TO STYLE NATURAL HAIR

HOW TO STYLE NATURAL HAIR

This is a big topic, and one that's hard to cover to include everyone properly. No matter how many I may share, there are several more to try. Natural hair is versatile. Much more than relaxed, even though I am not trying to look down on relaxed styles. I am merely sharing that you have more options, tools and looks you can rock with your own natural tresses.

There is a connection between wash day and styling. Washday is the foundation for your style so ensure hair is clean, properly moisturized, conditioned and ready for your styling product. Here are the most popular styles naturals wear and the products they use to create them:

- TWA (Teeny Weeny Afro)
- Twist outs & Flat Twist Out
- Braid Outs
- Bantu Knots (Outs)
- Flexi Rods
- Roller Sets
- Braids & Twists
- Finger Coils

- Straight Styles
- Buns
- Chignons
- Wash & Go
- Protective Styles (many on this list fall under this category)

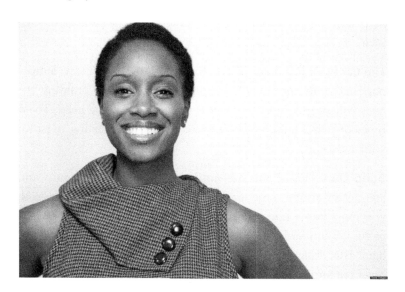

The beloved **TWA (Teeny Weeny Afro)** is a staple in the natural hair movement and is self-explanatory. Although hailed as an "Afro", the TWA is just short natural hair and usually the same length all the way around. It can be in any state of curl, kink or coil, and is the usual style most women start with after the Big Chop. This is one of the best short hairstyles to have fun with.

Twist Outs - One of the more popular hairstyles for naturals, the twist-out, allows for a uniform spiral or coil pattern in one's natural hair. This beautiful style can be done on hair as short as a TWA or as long as hair down to your hip bone. The twist-out is a protective style that also stretches hair and helps many naturals decrease problems with tangles. This win-win style requires you know how to twist one's own hair, either with two strands or three.

Simply place hair into twists and then unravel (once hair is completely dry) for your desired style. This can be achieved on fully wet hair (like right from washday) or on dry hair. Remember that product and some moisture should be added to help stave off dryness and frizz, while giving the style a polished look.

The **flat twist out** requires you to know how to cornrow. Simply part hair into cornrowed sections and instead of braiding the hair, you simply twist (flat twist) the hair down the head. These types of twists tend to give a more defined and lasting twist for your twist-out.

Braid Outs - Braid outs are similar to traditional twist outs and are created in the same manner, with some differences. First off, you must know how to braid. Secondly, this style tends to look better on kinkier hair; otherwise, expect more frizz on less kinky hair. This style also stretches the hair more than a traditional twist out and looks great on shorter hair.

Braid outs last longer when kept in braids longer and of course, starting out on freshly washed hair also allows this style to last longer. Expect more of a crimped look and less of a curlier look when doing braid outs.

Bantu Knot Outs - Bantu knots are a favorite among naturals, and they are excellent for transitioning naturals as well. What many often just think of roller sets or twist outs for getting a uniform curls, bantu knot outs do the very same thing and give a unique texture and style that lasts just as long and looks oh so amazing! There are two major ways to create your bantu knots.

For the first style, start off by applying a cream, gel or some sort of light holding products to the roots and strands, and carefully twists hair into the knot. You can twist in whatever direction you want, twist the hair into a knot and tuck the end under. If the ends can't stay put, you can choose to hold them down with a bobby pin. The second method gives your bantu knots an even curlier texture by twisting or braiding sections prior to creating your knot. You continue on just like the first method after that. You'd then take knots down once hair is dry and gently fluff so the style holds.

A newer alternative to roller sets that's very popular with naturals is the **Flexi Rods**. Best achieved on freshly washed hair (as most styles) flexi rods is a protective style that lasts as long as you care for it nightly and gives two or more very different textures a uniform and smooth look, on any hair type.

First, split your hair into sections for easier manageability. Take a square inch (or any small amount you prefer) of hair from each section, spritz with water and apply the leave-in conditioner. (This is exactly like applying setting lotion to hair when doing a roller set.) Brush to fully smooth hair and to disperse product. It will keep your hair stretched and detangled.

Now, place the end of your hair on the end of the flexi rod and wrap it around to secure it. Slowly roll the flexi rod and smooth the hair up to the root of the hair. Make sure to use the remainder of the flexi rod to close by bending it up to keep hair on the flexi rod and in place.

Repeat the process on the rest of your head, spritzing hair with water that may have dried slightly. When finished, you can air dry or use a hooded dryer, and then sleep with a satin bonnet. For the next day, make sure that your hair is 100% dry before you unravel each flexi rod (in an outward motion), slowly making sure not to disturb the curl pattern and cause frizz.

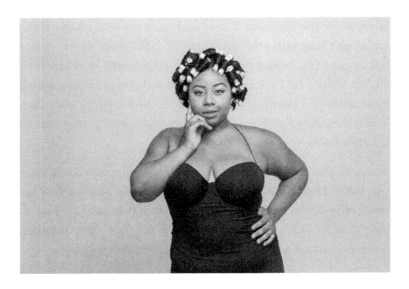

Roller sets are nothing new to black women. Often used to curl our chemically straightened hair for volume and body, roller sets serve more than one purpose for natural hair. Roller sets help to smooth, straighten and even create a uniform curls when hair is natural. Whether you choose to use magnetic rollers or perm rods, they both aid in the above-mentioned purposes and are great transitional styles.

Just like a flexi rod set, they are created best on freshly washed, still wet or damp hair. Hair should be completely free of tangles. Make sure to split your hair into sections for easier manageability, and take a square inch (or any small amount you prefer) of hair from each section and spritz with water and/ setting lotion mix. A good roller set relies on hair's tension on the roller to smooth out the curl. If your hair looks smooth and taut over the roller, then the hair will have a smooth finish. If not, then it can be frizzy and stretched but not with a smooth style.

Yes, the biggest problem you may face is fighting frizz and getting curls smooth. Practice certainly makes perfect but if you could create a mean roller set when relaxed, you will be able to do the same when natural, as long as you make sure to remove tangles and create damp, smooth hair on each roller. Always wait until hair is fully dry to take down or your curls will suffer.

Protective Styles are hairstyles that allow your hair to be protected from manipulation, styling, environment and clothing.

Here are some common protective styles:

- Mini Twists
- Weaves
- Senegalese twists
- Crochet braids
- Box Braids
- Goddess Braids
- Flat twists
- Cornrows
- Fish Tail Braids
- Faux locs

We will discuss protective styles in length in chapter 12.

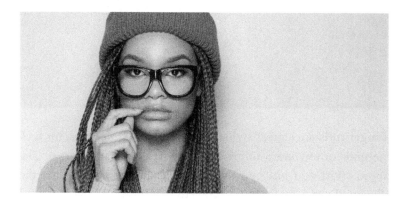

Braids & Twists are exactly what you think and are most often installed using braiding hair. If you are blessed with naturally thick hair, you can opt for just braiding and twisting your own hair, though the braiding hair helps the style last longer. These types of styles are considered protective styles, as long as you instill the tips mentioned above.

From box braids to crochet braids to senegalese twists, all of these types of styles last weeks or longer and are great for transitioners. They are also great for first-time naturals who are not really ready to deal with their own natural hair for styling just yet. As long as you cleanse, moisturize and protect your hair underneath, you are well on your way to a positive natural hair journey.

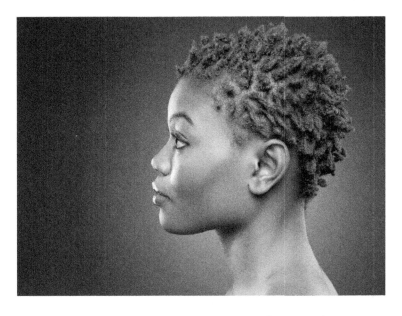

Finger coils are a great style for in-between hair lengths, for new naturals or anyone wanting a lasting style that looks great. The more effort you put into the style, the greater chance that the style will yield longer lasting coils that will keep all eyes on you! Great for short hair, finger coils give uniform coils on any hair length and texture. When completed on wash day, this style looks better as it ages.

Start on freshly washed and fully detangled hair. Hair also needs to stay very wet to coil properly, so have a spray bottle of water or setting lotion close by. Apply a leave-in all over and then section hair into small rows, while keeping all other hair clipped and out of the way. Add your choice of styling product that has a medium hold like a curling cream, mousse, setting lotion, or gel and part hair into rows. You can choose to not do that if you worry about spaces.

Twirl a three-inch section of hair around your finger, until it's tightly spiraled all the way down to the ends of your hair. Repeat until all of the hair is complete and seal your coils with an oil or balm of your choice. You can either air dry or sit under a dryer for hair to dry fully faster. The best part about this style is that is lasts at least a week or longer, and hair gets bigger and better as the style gets older.

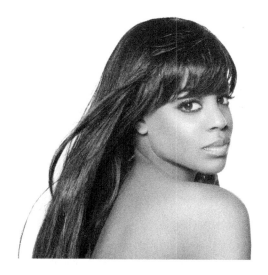

Straight Styles cause the most concern for new naturals because many get used to straight hair from their relaxed days and try and continue while natural. For one, your hair is different and will not be like straight hair when it was relaxed and two, bone straight hair can be very damaging to our natural strands. Opting for roller sets and then using a silk wrapping technique to achieve straight styles is a much healthier pathway to straight hair, but if you want to use heat-styling tools, there are smarter ways to do so and not jeopardize the health of your tresses.

Straight hair is a lovely option for many naturals, but it can be a dangerous process as it can damage the hair if not applied correctly or used too often. However, there is a way to not only stave off heat damage but to keep your strands healthy and moisturized. Top two tips to remember are to use only as high of a temperature as necessary and to pass through with the flat iron or hot comb ONCE.

Curlier, kinkier and *coilier* textures cannot withstand the high temperatures of heat appliances like naturally straight hair can, and many woman of color incur heat damage as a result. Heat damage is hair that has had heat-styling tools set on temperatures too high, too long, passed over too many times (or all of the above) and the hair loses its natural elasticity. This damages the hair shaft and changes the original curl, coil or kink.

Always start with fully cleansed hair. If using a heat-styling tool on dirty hair, you are searing all the product build-up, dirt and sweat into your strands. Your hair needs to be moisturized at the deepest level, and only certain ingredients have that ability to penetrate the hair shaft to do it. Make sure to concentrate on moisturizing fully by deep conditioning with heat. Moisturized hair just looks better and there's nothing worse than a straight style that looks brittle or dry. Heat protectants are necessary. They adhere to the strands like a shield and while keeping moisture in, they also protect the hair from the heat-styling tool. This will help keep your hair from drying out and allow you to use enough heat to make the style last longer.

Our hair LOVES water-based products but if you want your straight style to last longer, steer clear of them as they will make your hair revert back to its natural state. Also, avoid moisture at all costs by covering head with a scarf and plastic cap in the shower. If you work out, don't wrap up your hair if you sweat in your head. Place in a ponytail or up in a loose bun and allow to fully dry before wrapping at night.

I strongly advise (as do hairstylists) against wearing hair straight by using a flat iron, curling iron or hot comb too often. Even monthly is too often, honestly. Use these types of heat-styling tools sparingly as they can inflict heat damage with just one application and heat-styling tools that use direct heat can cause dryness to curlier textures.

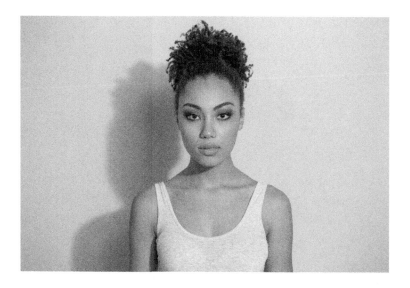

BUNS!! We love them, rock them and are forever finding new ways to give them life in our natural and curly hair. Buns are popular with natural and relaxed styles but with our natural texture, our buns have volume and character that straight hair just doesn't. A bun can be messy, to the back, up top, and even coupled with loose hair as the variations are pretty endless. Buns are not just for the medium to long-haired naturals as small buns or simply adding some hair can give you as big a bun as you dare. Think buns are boring? Check out all the cute ways to style them and see just how amazing this simple, yet fun, look gives your look. Check out the variety of buns that you can rock.

We love *messy buns*! They are the easiest of the sexiest and easiest curly hair bun styles to rock that allow you to look like you don't care while actually caring a lot! Usually up at the crown or top of your head, a messy bun is simply a haphazardly put together bun that is loose and has many of your coils, kinks and curls cascading about. When creating this style, think more of a carefree spirit than structure, and know that as long as you love it, the style will be great. Embrace your mass of textured hair and enjoy your messy bun.

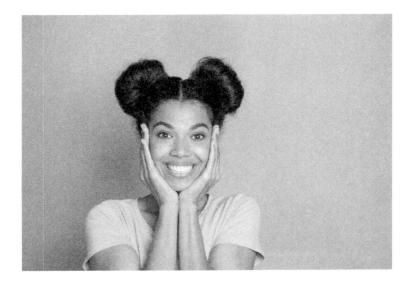

Space buns, afro puffs, double buns... However you care to call them, this style looks great on any curly-haired lovely. Whether they are side to side, or top and bottom, the double buns or space buns are all about having fun. Rules? What rules! They do not have to be even, nor on either side of your head. Don't forget the accessories that always look good in our hair like scarves and hair jewelry. Using hair extensions or braiding hair gives space buns height, width and even color so never feel limited by what you see others do. Do you and have fun with it.

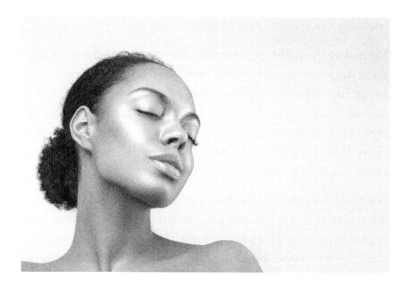

Chignons are quite popular for naturals as they exude elegance, softness and beauty. They are merely buns pinned into a knot at the nape of the neck or at the back of the head and often seen in wedding hair, many times accompanied by flowers. From twists to flowers, this lovely style is truly up to the creator and can be dressed up or down just as easily. This is an easy style to fake with added hair so don't feel left out TWAers! If you didn't notice, this is also a protective style that lasts and has an easy nighttime routine. Simply cover with a satin scarf or bonnet at night and slightly spritz down any flyaways in the morning. It's also a great style to wear from an older stretched style too.

It's hard to believe that I have to call this style, "old school." The **ninja bun or top knot** is simply a puff at the very top of your head, and the remaining hair loose is coming to a close. Just a few years ago, this style was ruling the natural hair movement and everyone was rocking one in varying ways. This is another great style to wear after an old twist/braid out or wash and go. Simply revive the curls with moisture, scrunching and a little gel. It will be good as new and give you a few more days until washday.

No matter the hair type, porosity or even length, the **wash-and-go** is simply wearing hair out with your very own hair texture. Every hair type is welcomed! The goal of a wash-and-go is to capture your own curl's definition. Moisture is key. Creating this style must start out on freshly washed and moisturized hair. There is no right or wrong look to the wash-and-go but all too often, this style is called the problem style.

For many naturals, the wash-and-go is hard to achieve, but more often than not, it is because you are not trying the various techniques to achieve the classic natural hairstyle. No one method is ideal for everyone, but the style is absolutely achievable by everyone! Many newly naturals find the wash-and-go easier on shorter hair, with less tangles to fight as a main perk.

I am a year round wash-and-go natural and have learned a few tips that make this style work well. My washday routine has to be on point. I cleanse well, moisturize, deep condition with heat, and apply my leave-in and gel to lock in moisture. When my washday is stellar, my wash-and-go lasts for days with me only having to lightly spritz and fluff in the morning. I have very tight coils and deal with a ton of shrinkage, but I love my wash-and-go. It's great for the lazy natural, in my book!

CHAPTER EIGHT

THE BALANCE BETWEEN MOISTURE & PROTEIN

Natural hair is delicate, but that doesn't mean we cannot find a healthy ground for it to thrive. What natural hair needs the most is a proper balance between moisture and protein. There is a co-dependent relationship between the moisture and protein contents in your strands. One cannot work without the other.

Our hair is made up of a very hard protein called Keratin. Quite often, that protein gets broken down by our manipulation, chemical processes, like color or relaxing, and the environment. Our hair also needs lots of moisture because that keeps our hair pliable and hydrated. Without that moisture, our hair becomes dry and brittle. When the hair is being moisturized, water molecules bind with the protein present in the strands. This is how they are able to absorb and perform hydrating duties.

If your hair care includes just moisturizing, the balance will be disturbed and your hair will not be in its healthiest state. Lack of this balance is the cause of many hair issues we spend hundreds of dollars trying to fix. Your hair care routines should be focused on keeping an equal balance between the moisture and protein content of your hair.

(Moisture + Protein = Healthy Hair)

To determine if you have the right balance, here's a quick and easy test you can do:

First, wet your hair thoroughly. By the way, water is the best moisturizer!

Next, pat dry with a microfiber towel. Never use a regular cotton bath towel.

And then, pull some strands, stretching them out without applying force on your scalp.

If your hair stretches slightly and bounces back to its original length without breaking, congratulations! You have balanced hair.

If your hair stretches too far and has a weak, spongy feel, that means it has too much moisture in it with no protein support. Improve your hair's protein level by using a protein building deep conditioner.

If your hair is hard and can't be managed, it usually means there's an overabundance of protein and too little moisture. If the hair hardly stretches and breaks off, you need to boost your moisture game. Hair like this is usually rough, tangled and brittle when dry. Start a moisturizing routine that includes a weekly moisturizing, deep conditioner treatment.

One of the best ways to incorporate moisture into your strands (and keep them in) is using the LCO or the LOC methods. They stand for:

LCO (Liquid + Cream + Oil) or LOC (Liquid + Oil + Cream)

This is merely the order you add these items to your hair to impart moisture into your hair and keep it sealed in. The liquid is almost always water and the cream is most often conditioner. The oil should be natural or a blend of oils. Either order is highly effective at keeping natural strands moisturized by applying the liquid, and then the cream and oil in either fashion. Water (or liquid) is always first but you can determine how to incorporate the last two, according to your preferences after trying both.

I moisturize a few days a week, but I know I must counter it with monthly or bi-monthly protein treatments to keep my hair strong. It may take a while to find your own perfect balance, but checking your hair will help you find it. I love wetting my hair in the shower and then sealing in that moisture with my favorite leave-in conditioner and oil that's been blended into a spray bottle. My blend is: distilled water, jojoba oil and lavender oil.

Now, let's discuss protein and whether or not you need protein in your routine? Protein in products improve the hair's elasticity and strength properties. Just as our bodies need this, our hair does as well. Taking heed to what it is and how to incorporate it into your hair care is important.

Now, how much and how often depends on what you are doing to your hair. Let's first talk about the different types of protein that can be used on our hair:

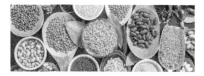

- Animal – Repairs damage to the outer layers of the hair.
- Collagen – Increases the elasticity of the hair.
- Silk – Tends to soften the hair.
- Vegetable – Can absorb more easily without leaving a build-up on the hair shaft and can attract moisture.

- Wheat – A moisturizing as well as strengthening protein. Also aids in maintaining moisture levels.

Milder applications of proteins are found in the shampoo and conditioner, and can be used weekly. Where you would find stronger amounts would be in protein treatments, and shouldn't be used as often. They should state on the products, "to be used every six to eight weeks." So, now let's see who needs just a regular 8 to 10 week treatment or more intense monthly treatment. If you do any of these things to your hair:

- Color
- Relax
- Texturize
- Heat style

You may need to have the more intense treatments. All of the above-mentioned can be damaging to your hair, but it doesn't mean you can't do them. It just means you need to understand that using or doing those things to your tresses requires more work in keeping the hair healthy.

WHAT IF YOU ARE PROTEIN-SENSITIVE?

Some feel they cannot use proteins or feel they are protein-sensitive. Suffering from protein-sensitivity simply means your hair responds negatively to the use of proteins like drying out, becoming brittle and even breaking off. One issue that may cause protein-sensitivity is using products with proteins too often. If using them sparingly and still suffering from these types of issues, then you might have true protein-sensitivity. All too often, women believe they are sensitive to ALL protein.To know for sure requires a simple test by wetting a section of hair, rubbing a protein ingredient on your sectioned hair and allowing the test patch to dry. If you notice negative effects like severe dryness or breakage, then you are more than likely sensitive to that particular protein.

You can try other types of proteins to see if your hair can tolerate another type, but make sure you are not overusing any products with protein. If you notice dry, brittle or broken strands of hair, be on alert. Many of our favorite brands and products, from gels to shampoos, use protein ingredients. So, if you are using them daily, you are over-processing your hair with protein and may be creating your own dryness and damage. This is why it is important to check the label on your products! Your hair will always be your best guide on when you hair needs some moisture, if it's too dry, or some protein, if it's too mushy. Pay attention and you will fare just fine.

CHAPTER NINE

DEFINITIONS - HAIR POROSITY & OTHER TERMS YOU NEVER KNEW

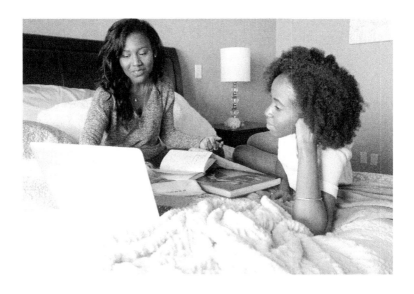

I never became more hair savvy until I went natural. I learned more about my hair than I ever knew when relaxed, and I shudder to think how little I knew about my hair when I used to regularly use harsh chemicals like relaxers. Now, I do not want to overwhelm you by scouring the internet and listing every natural hair term anyone has ever used. Instead, I will give you definitions on the most popular and useful terms that will allow you to fully understand what you need to know, whether relaxed or natural.

Every term may not apply to you or your hair, but they are popular for a reason as many naturals come across these terms.

2nd, 3rd, and 4th day hair – These are phrases used to describe the amount of time your hair has gone since you last heavily styled or manipulated it. Hair styled today would be considered 2nd day hair tomorrow. Light styling, like fluffing or spritzing with water, is usually done on 2nd, 3rd or even 4th day hair.

3a | 3b | 3c - These are classification numbers for naturally loose(r) curly hair. This hair system was created by Andre Walker, and is also called hair-typing. Most black women will fall under the 3c category, more often than 3a or 3b.

4a | 4b | 4c - These are classification numbers for naturally tight, kinky-curly hair. Most black women fall under the 3 and 4 hair category. Classification created by Andre Walker.

Accordion Technique (Method) - A squeezing motion, used to scrunch styling products into the strands of the hair, in order to encourage body and natural waves. The objective is to scrunch hair in the formation of an accordion.

Afro – **A** very popular natural hairstyle, often referred to as a "fro." This hairstyle is round in shape on naturally curly/coily hair.

Aloe Vera Juice/Gel - Conditions the hair while adding moisture and shine. It is also known for aiding in hair growth for people with hair loss. As a bonus, it's also excellent for detangling and soothing scalp irritation.

Alopecia – hair loss.

Alopecia Areata – An autoimmune disorder where an individual's immune system attacks their affected hair follicles and causes hair loss is patches. This is not contagious and is not caused by stress.

Almond Oil - This oil moisturizes and softens hair. Almond oil contains a large amount of Vitamin E and K along a host of other minerals such as calcium and magnesium. This makes almond oil one of the only oils that can prevent the hair from drying out and becoming brittle.

Amla Oil - It comes from Alma, botanically known as Amilica Embillicus. It's a small tree that is native to the Indian subcontinent. One of the most important plants in traditional Ayurvedic medicine, Amla has medicinal and anti-cariogenic properties. A natural powerhouse of goodness, it is rich in Vitamin C, Calcium, Phosphorus, Iron, Carotene, Vitamin B Complex and also a powerful antioxidant agent.

One of the most popular ways this oil is used for hair is as an after shampoo conditioner. This oil is great for decreasing hair fall, and increasing hair growth. With antifungal properties, this is an ideal oil to fight dandruff.

Amla Powder - Created by crushing dried amla. This powder gives cooler tones to red and brown henna hair dye. Henna lovers have been using Indigo to darken the red henna. So, when you add amla powder, you're creating an even cooler tone by preventing the indigo from fading and by reducing the red of the henna.

Amla oil brings back your normal curls and waves, which have been changed by henna. Many henna users have noticed a difference in their curls and waves as a result. Amla powder mixed in will tone down those changes. You'll notice more of your previous texture. Just like the oil, the powder is excellent for promoting healthy hair growth. You simply have to combine with an oil like coconut, to gain the benefits. One of the best ways is a super easy hair mask.

APL (Armpit Length) - Refers to hair that reaches the armpit. So, it's essentially a hair length term.

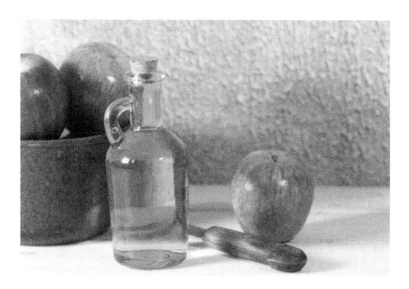

Apple Cider Vinegar (ACV) - This product is useful for clarifying hair from build-up, helps to seal ends after shampooing, and eliminates dandruff. ACV corrects the pH balance of hair, aids in closing the hair's cuticle so strands are smooth with less frizz. It's also great as a base for some DIY hair mixes.

Apricot Oil - This oil is derived from dried apricot kernels (Prunus armeniaca) that have been cold-pressed or through solvent extraction. Apricot oil is an emollient that has anti-inflammatory, anti-aging, anti-bacterial, antiseptic and antioxidant properties. Apricot oil is very light, and therefore allows it to be used as a sealant, leave-in, pre-poo, post-poo, hot oil treatment, and treatment for dry scalp. Apricot oil seals moisture into the hair shaft by shaping the scales of the cuticle and holding them together.

Argan Oil - This oil is derived from the argan tree nuts of the native Argan tree in Morocco. Known as "liquid gold," this oil has been used as a skin moisturizer and hair conditioner since ancient times. Argan oil has a unique composition with more than 200% tocopherols (vitamin E) than olive oil and very high levels of fatty acids. Argan oil has Squalene, Polyphenols and Sterols. It's excellent for protecting hair while swimming, as it won't weight hair down. It further helps to restore hair's shine and softness, while preventing dryness.

Avocado Oil - Rich in potassium, vitamin E, protein, vitamin A, vitamin K, fiber, folate, vitamin B6, vitamin C and protein, avocado oil is a natural hair and skin healer. Since it is close to the natural composition of the oils our skin naturally produce, it is easily absorbed and able to aid in healing. This is great when dealing with rough, cracked skin. Avocado oil also contains anti-fungal and anti-bacterial properties vital when treating skin conditions, such as eczema or psoriasis, that may flare up during the winter.

The fatty richness of avocado is good for healing, moisturizing, and protecting the hair as it contains most of the nutrients and vitamins produced in our sebum. Because of this fact, the oil is absorbed easily into the hair and scalp. It seals in moisture and protects the hair from the elements. From deep conditioning masks to hot oil treatments, the fats that the avocado contains have proven to provide not only moisture, but essential nutrients and vitamins that enable healthy hair growth and repair damage.

Ayurvedic Regimen - Inspired by traditional Indian practices, this regimen emphasizes the use of plant extracts like amla oil, neem, and henna to encourage the growth of strong hair.

Baggy Method - Helps to reduce breakage, split ends, and dryness. After moisturizing your hair and sealing it at night, put a plastic cap or shower cap on overnight to help your hair retain the moisture it needs for maximum growth retention and softness.

Banding - The banding method is a 'shrink fighting,' or shrinkage fighting, natural hair technique. Simply put, place sectioned hair in ponytails, scrunchies, or hair ties to allow hair to dry while stretching.

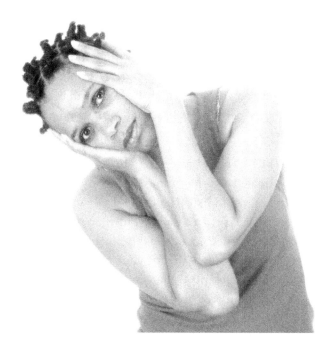

Bantu Knots - Bantu knots have a rich history in African culture and are by no means ever called or seen as "mini buns". These beautiful coils are not knots at all but buns of sectioned hair, twisted and secured against the side of the head. You can create the Bantu knot-out on stretched hair or even on two (or more) different textures of relaxed and natural hair. The knots create a curvy, coily set to the hair, allowing you to mask the difference in textures and look like you are all natural. Relaxed hair tends to be limp and lack structure so this style gives life back to those strands.

Bantu Knot-Out - Simply create the style as suggested above, unravel the bantu knots and fluff. Make sure hair is completely dry prior to unraveling the knots or twists. This is a great style for transitioners who want a uniform curl on relaxed or natural hair.

Baobab oil - Extracted from the seeds of the Adansonia tree, Baobab oil is one of the most prominent oils in Africa and is becoming increasingly popular among naturals. This ultra-light oil is an emollient and rejuvenator that moisturizes without weighing down hair. Baobab oil is great for hot oil treatments, and is a light sealant that will add sheen without making hair greasy. Another perk, baobab oil will protect hair from the sun and tame frizz.

Big Chop (BC) - This phrase refers to cutting off all relaxed or chemically treated strands immediately, or starting fresh with only natural or virgin hair. The method allows you to use products for one hair type, and most women are left with a TWA or Teeny Weeny Afro. Understandably, this may be a daunting prospect if you have never worn your hair cropped before, but many ladies have described the experience as freeing. So if you are brave and impulsive, this is the path for you. Doing the Big Chop (BC) can be done by you or a professional, especially if you are looking for a style.

Bentonite Clay - Bentonite clay is composed of aged, volcanic ash, and can draw-out toxins from the body. It has an abundance of minerals, including calcium, magnesium, silica, sodium, copper, iron and potassium.

Biotin - Also known as vitamin B7, it is used by the body to metabolize carbohydrates, fats and amino acids. It is a highly popular vitamin for hair, skin and nails and can be taken as a supplement alone, or in a multivitamin, most often labeled as a hair, skin or nail vitamin. Biotin strengthens the actual hair follicles and this water-soluble vitamin helps produce healthy hair proteins like Keratin.

Box Braids - This is a protective hairstyle usually created with braiding. The hair is placed into individual plaits that are usually divided by small, squared off parts or boxes. The braiding hair gets wrapped around the roots of each section and woven down to halfway or all the way to the tip.

Braid Out - This hairstyle is achieved by braiding sections of damp or moist hair and unraveling once it is dry. The hair will have more defined curls or waves. This style is also popular with transitioners and helps to stretch the hair.

Brazilian Keratin Treatment / Brazilian Blowout / Keratin Treatment - A chemical blowout treatment used to temporarily smooth and straighten natural, textured hair. This method of temporarily straightening hair uses a flat iron to trap a liquid keratin and preservative solution into the hair shaft. The effects only last around three months but there has been some concerns over the ingredients in the solution and its effect on the workers in salons as well as the wearer. The object is to keep hair frizz-free or straight for a few months, and there are some at-home kits.

BSL (Bra Strap Length) - Refers to hair that reaches the bra strap on your back. It's a hair length term.

Buds (Budding) - First stage of dreadlocks (locs), when a knot is formed as the nucleus of each lock.

Butters (hair butters, natural butters) - Butters are natural blends of organic oils and unrefined butter that acts as moisturizing sealants to protect hair from dryness and breakage. Butters can be mixtures that contains natural butters, such as mango and cocoa, and oils, such as olive and coconut. Butters are thick, which allows them to really coat, protect, and remain present on the hair strands longer than just using oils. They also offer a variety of vitamins and nutrients to the hair, which are important factors when dealing with harsh temperature changes.

Caffeine - This substance stimulates our Central Nervous System and can be found in over 60 plants. Now, while the FDA DOES classify caffeine as a drug and food additive, did you know it also encourages hair growth? Caffeine can interact with the hair follicles, even regulating and promoting hair growth, while thwarting hair loss.

Camellia Oil - An amazing oil that's full of hair-loving fatty acids, this carrier oil has properties to condition hair while unblocking pores to the scalp. It stimulates hair growth and controls water loss in hair. It also contains Omega-9 or oleic acid, which will make your strands softer and more pliable. Camellia oil also has stearic acid, which is excellent for protecting and conditioning tresses while palmitic acid adds moisture to the hair.

Canopy - Represents all the hair that is on the outskirts of your hairline, mostly at the top of your head. This section of hair is more prone to frizz because it's bombarded by the elements from the sun, wind, rain and even pollutants.

Carrier Oils - Known as base oils, they are often used to dilute essential oils(EO). They are thicker, fatty oils derived from plants and therefore, have many therapeutic properties. Several have huge benefits on the hair and scalp. Popular examples are: Coconut, Shea and Olive.

Castor Oil - Castor oil is a natural oil that is rich in fatty acids and other nutrients that help to moisturize, strengthen and condition the hair. It's best known for having the amazing ability to promote growth in all hair types. It contains hair growth and regeneration properties. The oil's triglycerides of ricinoleic acid makes it anti-fungal, anti-bacterial and anti-inflammatory. This further makes it an ideal oil for combating and preventing scalp infections, fungi and unhealthy bacteria.

Cayenne Pepper - Cayenne pepper has anti-inflammatory, anti-allergen, anti-fungal and anti-irritant properties. It also contains vitamin A, vitamin B6, vitamin C, beta-carotene, manganese and potassium. While all are amazing for our bodies, these properties are great for stopping hair loss and promoting hair growth.

In a nutshell, the capsaicin in cayenne pepper stimulates hair growth by promoting blood circulation to the hair follicles, which ensures better nutrition. Capsaicin also stimulates dormant hair follicles, thus helping the volume and thickness. If that's not enough, it can even add some sheen and softness to your tresses.

CBL (Collar Bone Length) - A hair length term, it refers to hair that reaches the collar bone.

CG / CGM - Short for "curly girl" or "curly girl method." The Curly Girl Method is a revolutionary method of caring for curly hair, from the tightest to loosest in the book "Curly Girl," written by Lorraine Massey and Michele Bender. Many consider it the curly girl's bible.

Chunky Fro – This represents a hairstyle where the hair is set in a chunky twist style then unraveled. The goal is to have the unraveled twists show texture and stand up/out, considering it a newer version of the Afro. It is not your average rounded afro as this hair resembles chunks.

Clarifying Shampoo - A clarifying shampoo is an ultra-cleansing shampoo that remove all traces of dirt and product build-up. It is needed for removing hard-water deposits and chlorine.

Clumping - This condition is created when strands of hair collect in groups to form a more defined curl or wave. It's a desired effect in natural hair styling.

Coconut Oil - This is the extracted oil from the fruit (coconut) of the coconut tree. It's an edible oil, consumed in tropical places for thousands of years. Coconut benefits our bodies from inside to out and despite what most know about this oil, there is more than just one type.

Unrefined (virgin) coconut oil – retains the original coconut's chemical composition, which is made from fresh coconut meat and considered superior to the other two forms.

Refined coconut oil – is made from dried coconut meat that has been bleached, deodorized, treated and processed through high temperatures extract flavor and aroma.

While some nutrients are stripped the fatty acid composition is untouched.

Fractionated coconut oil – Most are unaware of this type that stays in liquid form and is only a fraction of coconut oil. Just about all the long, chain triglycerides are removed through hydrolysis and steam distillation. Coconut oil is rich in carbohydrates, vitamins and minerals. For a long time, it was demonized by high saturated fat content. People are beginning to think differently about this oil as those saturated fats are handled differently in our bodies. It contains healthy fats or good fats called medium-chain fatty acids (MCFAs) like Caprylic acid, Lauric acid and Capric acid.

Cold-Pressed - Represents an ideal method of extracting oils and butters from seeds, using friction to help keep the important properties intact. The temperature of the seeds never exceed 49 °C (120 °F), thus enabling them to retain their nutrients and natural scents.

Coils - groups of small, spring-like curls.

Collagen Protein - Collagen is a protein our bodies naturally produce and is pretty much the glue that holds our bodies together. It gives our skin and hair strength, elasticity and actually helps to replace dead skin cells. Collagen directly and positively affects hair growth through hair regeneration. This keeps hair strong, fights off free radicals and improves hair volume by increasing the diameter of each individual hair, giving a fuller look.

Comb coils - A natural hairstyle achieved by placing the tail of a rattail comb at the root of small sections of the hair and turning clockwise to create a coil.

Cones (Silicones) - Silicones are plastic-like polymers that are used in hair products to lubricate, condition and add shine. They are usually identified by names that end in "-cone," "col," "conol," or "-zane," which makes them easy to spot on product labels. Typically, silicones are used to coat the hair shaft in order to prevent frizz, smooth the cuticle and protect against thermal damage from heat-styling tools. The two most common forms of silicones are non-soluble and water soluble.

Co-Wash - A co-wash or co-washing is the same as washing with shampoo, but replaced with conditioner. Shampoo is deeply cleansing the hair, and can harm and strip the hair of essential oils. Shampooing too often is actually not good for our curly strands, but do not completely remove it from your regimen. A co-wash can cut down on how often a natural needs to shampoo and since it mildly cleanses the hair, some naturals have stopped using shampoo altogether. This is a term stemming from the Curly Girl Method.

Creamy Crack - A negative term to describe chemical relaxers.

Crochet Braids - Method of adding extensions to one's hair. The basis of the method is first cornrowing and then applying the extensions to the cornrows. The hair used is loose and not on a weft. Hair is looped under the cornrows with a crochet needle and secured with a crochet knot. Crochet braids can be long, short, straight, curly, blond or every other color on the color wheel. The styles are so amazing that often, many will never even know you are wearing them. Crochet braids don't last as long as other braids or twists but are often cheaper, more versatile and a much quicker install.

Crunch (Gel Cast) - the tough and crusty texture of dried up gel on your strands once hair is dry. Simply rub a light oil on hands and scrunch the hair. This removes the gel cast.

Curl Pattern - the looseness or tightness of your curls.

Deep Condition (DC) - A wash day treatment to protect and moisturize hair. A deep conditioning product is applied to freshly washed hair and kept in for at least 15 minutes as the product penetrates the hair shaft. It works better with heat, like a heating cap or hooded dryer.

Deep Conditioner - Deep conditioners are penetrating conditioners that add moisture, maintain elasticity, and strengthen the hair strands on a deeper level. They actually penetrate the hair shaft, though not all products have that ability. That's the magic behind a deep conditioner and why they are necessary on every single washday. They are necessary to not only protect and keep hair moisturized but to also combat the damages inflicted on your hair during washing, styling and regular day to day wear.

Detangle (detangling) - Natural hair is not straight so it coils and curls around itself. This causes tangles and snags. The act of removing those tangles is called detangling or to detangle. You can use fingers, wide tooth combs, detangling tools or even detangling hair products to aid. Detangling is most often done on wash day.

Diffuser - Hair diffusers are blow dryer attachments that disperses airflow over a large area. This design allows the attachment to aid in drying without disturbing the curl pattern or causing frizz. One of the best things about diffusers is the fact that they add volume and body, which is great for those of us with fine hair.

The benefits of using a diffuser includes: maximized shine, decreased frizz, enhanced curls, increased volume, minimized heat exposure and most importantly, hair that is dried quickly but gently.

Dreadlocks / Dreads / Locs - twisted and matted ropes of hair. They can form naturally through the matting process when hair is not brushed or combed, or intentionally formed with combs and locking products.

Dusting - This is a trimming technique where you take off such a small amount of your ends that it looks like dust on the floor, hence the name. It's a much smaller amount compared to a regular trim, since you are taking off about 1/4 of an inch. This is a great way to fight off split ends before they start. This is usually done at home and every 6 to 8 weeks, if needed. Make sure to use the proper shears!

Elasticity - This refers to the ability of your strands to stretch and bounce back without breaking. Healthy hair can be stretched completely straight, and bounces back to the original coil without breaking.

Emu Oil - Emu oil is obtained from the fat of the Emu bird (found in Australia) and collected mainly from the back and the rump. The benefits are amazingly extensive from cell growth to anti-inflammatory properties.

EO (Essential Oils) - Contraction of the original "quintessential oil", essential oils are naturally occurring, volatile aromatic compounds found in the bark, flowers, roots, seeds, stems and other parts of plants. When introduced in hair, they are often diluted with a carrier oil or even water. Several of them, like lavender or tea tree oil, are excellent for hair and scalp.

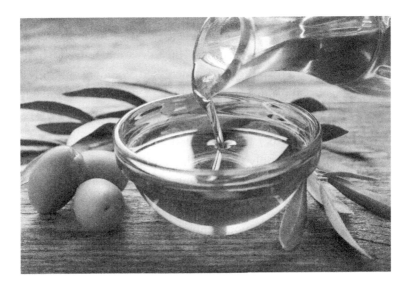

EVOO (Extra Virgin Olive Oil) - Extra-virgin olive oil is an unrefined oil and the highest-quality you can use. (See **Olive Oil** for more.)

Finger Coils - Finger coils give uniform coils on any hair length and hair texture. Popular on short-haired naturals, they're just sections of hair that are repeatedly twisted around one's finger to produce individual coils. Some may use a rat tail comb instead of their finger.

Flat Twist (Out) - Creating flat twists are not as difficult as creating cornrows. They use two strands of hair instead of three. Hair needs to be fully detangled. This style is best done on fully stretched hair (if you have 4C) or on freshly washed. Hair is placed into cornrowed sections; instead of braiding (as you would for cornrows) and for better definition, coil the individual strands before twisting them around one another. To wear out, simply unravel when dry.

Flax Seed Gel - Flax Seeds are rich in micronutrients, fiber, manganese, and essential fatty acid omega-3. When turned into an easy DIY gel, it has numerous benefits for natural hair. It leaves hair soft, shiny, and moisturized, while promote hair growth. The gel is excellent for curl definition, leaves no crunch, dries fast and gives hair a lot of slip.

Flexi Rods (Set) - Flexi Rods are flexible, long rollers that create sleek spiral curls on all hair textures. They come in different sizes to give varying curls and widths, and are easy to use. They are great for transitioners.

Fluff - The use of fingers or a pick to add volume and shape to natural hair. It also describes how many style hair on 2nd, 3rd or 4th day.

Fractionated Coconut Oil – Most are unaware of this type of coconut oil. It remains in liquid form and is only a fraction of coconut oil. Just about all the long chain triglycerides are removed through hydrolysis and steam distillation.

Frizz - A natural's sworn enemy, frizz is dehydrated strands. This occurs when the cuticle layer of your hair is raised, which allows moisture to pass through and swell the strand.

Frohawk - A natural (and better) take on the mohawk, this hair-style has the sides of an afro flattened to the scalp, either by smoothing & pinning, or by shaving. The center hair is left high and free, in the shape of the distinct Mohawk.

Garlic Oil - Garlic oil contains essential elements including sulfur, copper, vitamin C, selenium, and minerals that are highly beneficial for hair growth. Garlic has anti-microbial, anti-fungal, and antibiotic properties. It is said to stimulate blood flow to the scalp, in turn, encourages hair growth. You can add it to your shampoo or conditioner, use it in a scalp massage with another oil or for a hair massage all by itself.

Ginger - This root is part of the Zingiberaceae family, along with cardamom and turmeric. It is commonly produced in India, Jamaica, Fiji, Indonesia, and Australia. Ginger actually has a range of benefits for the scalp, roots and ends of hair, from stopping thinning to increasing blood flow, and giving the hair much needed minerals.

Going Natural - Common term for letting relaxed hair grow out so you can enjoy your natural hair texture. You can either chop it all of with a Big Chop or work with both textures for a longer period of time called Transitioning.

Grapeseed Oil - Grapeseed oil is one of the lightest oils available and much cheaper than Argan oil. Extracted from wine grapes, this oil has a great composition of fatty acids and properties, like vitamin E. Grapeseed oil has antioxidant and anti-inflammatory benefits, which makes it ideal for conditioning and moisturizing the hair and scalp.

Odorless and ultra-light, grapeseed oil is an excellent natural heat protectant and very close in composition as jojoba oil, which is very close to human sebum. Its rich, silky texture is perfect for soothing away dryness and irritation, and is suitable for all skin types since it won't clog pores or cause breakouts.

Growth Cycle - Hair grows in cycles: Anagen is the active phase, Catagen phase is a transitional stage, Exogen is the shedding phase and Telogen is the resting phase.

Hair Cuticle – the outermost layer of the hair. The cuticle tends to be unorganized and overlapping like a roof shingle, and these layers work defensively to prevent damage to the hair's innermost structure while holding onto the water content of the hair fiber. The strongest hair has a smooth, closed cuticle because when the cuticle is raised or chipped, it is extremely difficult to maintain moisture levels.

Hair Density - refers to how tightly the individual strands of hair are packed together on your head. The average person has around 2,200 strands of hair per square inch.

Hair Elasticity – is the ability of your strands to stretch and bounce back without breaking. Healthy hair can be stretched completely straight and bounce back to its original coil without breaking.

Hair Porosity – Porosity refers to how well your hair absorbs and holds moisture. Hair porosity is one of the main culprits that may hinder your attempts at maintaining or increasing your hair's moisture content. Think of your hair strands as covered in 'scales.' These "scales' allow water (moisture) into your strands. There are three types: Low, Medium and High.

Hair Types - Hair-typing is an easy way to determine what type of curls you have. Although it is obvious enough that natural hair varies in texture, hair-typing is a system that makes it easy to point out what category your strands fall in. There are several hair-typing systems, but the most popular one was created by hair stylist Andre Walker. The Andre Walker system divides hair into these categories: type 1- straight hair, type 2- wavy hair, type 3- curly hair and type 4- kinky hair. Each category also has sub-categories that divide them into different segments, depending on texture and curl pattern.

Hands In Hair - a made up term to describe naturals who cannot stop touching their hair. This action can cause frizz and/or damage if done excessively.

Havana Twists - Very similar to Marley Twists, Havana Twists are much larger than Marley Twists. Havana Twists are thicker, fuller twists with just two strands. Havana hair twists use Havana hair extensions.

Heat Damage - Heat damage is hair that has had heat-styling tools set on temperatures too high, too long, passed over too many times (or all of the above), and the hair loses its natural elasticity. This damages the hair shaft and changes its original curl, coil or kink. Heat damage is irreversible AND there is no such thing as heat training. If your hair does not revert back to it's natural coil, kink or coil, it has incurred heat damage.

Heat Training - *There is no such thing as heat training,* but many naturals think if they break the bonds of their hair with heat that this keeps the hair from reverting. All this is, is heat damage. *Heat training DOES NOT EXIST* and if you hair does not revert back to its natural texture, you have heat damage.

Hemp Seed Oil - Hemp seed oil is pressed from the seeds of the Cannabis sativa plant and contains 80% essential fatty acids. Hemp seed oil is excellent for skin and hair. It's an excellent conditioning agent and strengthens the hair structure.

Henna - Henna is a natural, reddish-brown dye that comes from the powdered leaves of a tropical plant that grows in the hot and dry climates of the Eastern hemisphere. It can be used to color hair (and/or decorate the body). Naturals use it because it's safer than traditional dyes. Users can get different variations of red, depending on where it was grown and ranging from auburn to cherry. Henna is known to highlight your hair. Also, after using henna, your hair is stronger, shinier and healthier because it fills in the weak areas of the hair strand; hence, it's a great conditioning treatment.

It seems that henna changes the weight of the strands through plant deposits, although it does not change the chemical structure of the strand. Henna also fills in rough spots on the cuticle, while makeing hair softer and smoother for many who use it.

High Porosity (hair) - Porosity refers to how well your hair absorbs and holds moisture. High porosity hair has the main issue of moisture retention. This hair type absorbs moisture readily, but loses it just as quickly. High porosity can be either a genetic property of hair or a result of damage from chemical processing or manipulation. There are gaps and holes in the cuticle, which may lead to too much moisture into the hair, and that also escapes just as easily.

Honey - Honey, a natural humectant and moisturizer, is a sweet food made by bees from the flower's nectar. It contains enzymes, vitamins, minerals, water and pinocembrin. Honey is an emollient so it not only seals in moisture, but also helps to condition your strands.

Humectants – refers to any substance that captures from surrounding air into the hair shaft. Products that have humectant properties are essential for maintaining natural hair.

Indigo - Indigo powder is from the ground leaves of the indigo plant. It contains a dark blue dye used for centuries in textiles but is an excellent source as a natural hair colorant. Many naturals use indigo in conjunction with henna to get a darker color as henna turns hair red.

Jamaican Black Castor Oil - Extracted differently from regular castor oil, Jamaican Black Castor Oil is processed traditionally and loaded with vitamin E, omega-6 and omega-9 fatty acids. These nutrients help moisturize hair while staving off breakage and even encouraging hair growth. Brown in color and thick, this favorite among naturals is often used for regrowing thinning edges and sealing ends.

Jojoba Oil - Not really an oil at all, but instead a liquid wax extracted from the nut of an indigenous American shrub, it goes by the scientific name Simmondsia chinensis. It's closest to our body's natural oil sebum, which makes it great for all skin types and therefore a natural skin conditioner. Jojoba oil controls hair loss by helping the follicles grow new hair, and moisturize dry and frizzy strands.

Kaolin Clay - Kaolin clay is a naturally occurring clay mostly found in soils developed from the hot, moist climates. Other than detoxing your hair of chemicals and pollutants, kaolin clay is an excellent choice for dry, brittle hair. Whether your hair is in this condition because of tap water, chemical processing or continued use of chemical hair products, you can use this to help restore the moisture.

Keratin - 90% of your hair is made up of keratin. It is a strong protein, formed by the combination of 18 amino acids. Keratin is the key structural building block of hair, skin, and nails, and while strong, it is still vulnerable to damage.

Kokum Butter - is derived from the Kokum fruit of the Garcina Indica tree. Native to the western ghat region of India, Kokum butter looks similar to shea butter, but contains a mild, almost non-existent scent. This butter is rich in antioxidants, vitamin E, citric acid, and essential fatty acids which makes it a great butter to soothe dry, itchy scalp. One of the best things about this oil is the fact that it's non-comedogenic, meaning it doesn't clog your pores or hair follicles. The vitamins and nutrients in the butter are better absorbed by the scalp and hair, which will promote healthier hair growth.

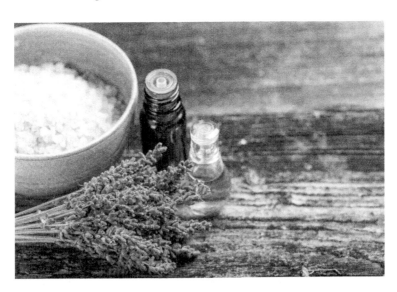

Lavender Oil - Lavender oil is extracted from the flowers of the lavender plant through steam distillation. Lavender oil is stimulating and in turn, increases circulation to the scalp. Lavender oil encourages new hair growth, provides much needed nutrients and oxygen to the root of the hair, and makes the root stronger. This reduces the amount of hair shedding.

Leave-in Conditioner - Leave-in's are light, water-based conditioners that have been specially formulated to allow for more frequent use than regular rinse-out conditioners. Leave-in conditioners don't require rinsing and can be used daily without excessive build-up. Many leave-in conditioners contain humectants, which draw water into the hair. This makes leave-in conditioners perfect for moisturizing and preventing dryness. Basically, using a leave-in protects and hydrates your hair for lasting moisture and style.

Length Retention - refers to holding onto your hair longer. That means caring or keeping the oldest hairs (the ends) in better condition and healthier.

LCO - A Liquid + Cream + Oil application to retain moisture in natural hair. There are two methods: the LOC or the LCO. Either is highly effective at keeping natural strands moisturized by applying the liquid, and then the cream and oil in either fashion.

Line of Demarcation - is the hair or the point of hair that separates the two textures of natural and relaxed for a new natural. This hair is weak. Because of it's fragile nature, being gentle is a must and using the correct tools will lower your breakage. Using wide tooth combs, Denman brushes (a popular brand of natural hair brushes) or your fingers when manipulating the hair is best. Also, low manipulation styles are recommended. This hair is the reason many decide on doing a BC as working with two textures can be difficult, though it CAN be done.

LOC - is a Liquid + Oil + Cream application to retain moisture in natural hair. There are two methods: the LOC or the LCO. Either method is highly effective at keeping natural strands moisturized by applying the liquid, and then the cream and oil in either fashion.

Low Porosity (hair) - Porosity refers to how well your hair absorbs and holds moisture. With low porosity, your hair has a tightly bound cuticle layer which pretty much repels water. You may notice that your hair takes a longer time to feel wet during the washing process and a longer time to dry.

MBL (Middle Back Length) - hair that can stretch just past one's bra strap. A hair length term.

Macadamia Nut Oil - comes from macadamia nuts, which have a rich flavor and are very high in nutrients. Excellent for skin and hair, Macadamia Nut Oil increases shine and improves the health of your hair. It strengthen the hair follicles and in turn, combats hair loss.

Mango Butter - The second most popular butter in the natural hair community is mango butter. Originated from Southern Asia, mango butter is extracted from the kernels of the mango and contains very high levels of antioxidants and vitamins. Having very similar qualities and benefits as Shea, mango butter soothes, protects, and seals, in addition to conditioning.

Since mango butter contains higher levels of fatty acids, it aids in conditioning the hair more thoroughly than Shea. Its high levels of vitamins A and C have also been shown to accelerate cell reproduction, which will result in a healthier scalp and promote hair growth.

Marley Twists/Kinky Twists - Smaller than Havana Twists, Marley Twists are two-strand twists with using Marley braiding hair. They are thinner and smoother than Havana Twists.

Marshmallow Root - A herb that's been around for centuries,

Marshmallow Root extract contains flavonoids, and has anti-inflammatory properties. Naturals are primarily using marshmallow root to detangle. Since the mucous-like consistency of marshmallow root is similar to flax seed and Aloe Vera gel, it makes the hair very slippery and easy to detangle.

Marula Oil - Made from the fruit of the marula tree, native to Africa, Marula Oil has high levels of vitamin C and oleic acid. This beauty oil contains 60% higher antioxidants concentration than the Argan oil and protects hair against environmental elements and harmful UV rays. It's a high moisturizing oil that's excellent for frizzy hair.

Medium Porosity (hair) - Porosity refers to how well your hair absorbs and holds moisture. For medium porosity, the cuticle layer is looser which allows just the right amount of moisture to enter while also preventing too much from escaping. Normal porosity hair holds styles well. Chemical manipulation, like color and relaxers, work well on this hair type.

Moisturize - Moisture is extremely important for natural hair's health. Unfortunately, the kinkier or coilier your hair is, the drier it can be. Moisturizing should be a vital component in your hair care regimen. Keeping natural hair moisturized is imperative for healthy and beautiful hair. Our tresses require more protection, natural oils and moisture to keep hair from getting brittle and damaged. Too often, newbies assume that slathering hair with any old oil or hair grease will moisturize hair but in reality, only a few natural oils are moisturizing oils.

Good old-fashioned water is the best and simplest moisturizer on the planet. Natural hair needs water to maintain its elasticity or the ability to stretch. It nourishes our strands and many products, if not the majority for our strands, have water as the very first ingredient.

Murumuru Butter - Native to the Amazon Rainforest in Brazil, this butter is extracted from the seeds of a fruit that grows on the Astrocaryum murumuru tree. This butter pretty much works like any other butter which promotes moisture retention, restores sheen and softens the hair.

Mustard Oil - This very popular oil of the Indian Subcontinent is either extracted by cold compression of mustard seeds or from steam distillation of mustard seeds soaked in water. The essential oil has the purpose of massage, and will also stimulates circulation, though best if not consumed orally. Mustard oil has antibacterial and anti-fungal properties, but it is becoming known as a hair revitalizer. With the oleic and Linoleic fatty acids, it has stimulating effects that increase blood circulation to the scalp which nourishes the hair follicles and encourages hair growth.

Neem Oil - comes from the large green tree and has been used in India since 2000-4000 BC. This oil is naturally yellow to brown in color and has a bitter taste with a garlic/sulfur smell. Extracted from the seeds and fruits of the neem tree, neem oil is a natural insect repellent. It contains antioxidants that help in fighting free radicals or UV rays. It also takes care of the blood vessels and cells of the scalp; as a result, normal hair growth is initiated.

The fatty acids of neem oil, like linoleic, oleic, stearic, act as an excellent conditioner for the hair and scalp. They nourish the hair and the scalp. These fatty acids help retain moisture on your hair and scalp and as a result, curb the dry and dullness of hair. If your hair is undernourished and rough, regular use of neem oil is sure to give your hair a shiny and healthy glow.

No-Poo - A non-foaming, non-detergent cleanser; it's usually a botanical conditioner, used to remove dirt, oils, environmental pollutants and styling products from the hair and scalp. It's less harsh on natural coils, curls and kinks.

Non-Soluble Silicones - These silicones cannot be removed or penetrated with water, which can be inadvertently damaging to the hair. These silicones can only be removed from the hair shaft by washing with clarifying shampoos or shampoos with harsh sulfates. These types of shampoos, although sometimes necessary, are drying to the strands. The problem with non-soluble silicones is the fact that they seal completely, allowing no moisture to penetrate the hair shaft until the silicone is washed out.

This causes hair to become dry and brittle, leading to damage and breakage. Non-soluble silicones should be avoided, especially for us curly/coily hair-types. The one good thing about them is that they work to prevent reversion and thermal damage if you're considering straightening your hair. If you do choose to use non-soluble silicones, then be sure to thoroughly cleanse the hair at least once a week and follow up with a deep conditioner so that the strands do not become dehydrated. Some non-soluble silicones that are typically found in hair products include: Behenoxy dimethicone, Cyclomethicone, Dimethicone, Trimethylsilyamodimethicone, Dimethiconol, and Cyclotetasiloxane.

Oil Rinsing - Consists of using oil in your wash day routine to aid in moisture retention, and remove knots and tangles. Some use this as a cleanser instead of shampoo. Others use oil rinsing after washing hair to combat the harshness of shampoos on natural hair.

Olive Oil - Aside from being great for cooking, olive oil has a lot of amazing benefits for skin and hair. Packed full of vitamins E and A, olive oil has amazing anti-aging properties, treats inflammation, acne, and also aids in the moisturization of excessively dry skin and hair. This oil has the power to both regenerate skin cells and help improve the elasticity of the skin. The best way to reap the full benefits of its anti-aging properties is to apply a small amount of olive oil to your skin before heading to bed on a daily basis.

In addition to that, olive oil also promotes hair growth, acts as a natural conditioner, imparts shine and treats itchy scalp and dandruff, which is especially important to keep in mind during the winter months. Due to its thick nature, olive oil is a great component to add to your hair care regimen, if you're looking to protect your hair from the harsh, cold climate.

Parts of the hair strand - Root (part growing in the follicle), Shaft (middle of the length of the hair), Tip (the end of the hair farthest away from the root).

There are also three layers to hair: the Medulla (innermost layer of the hair), the Cortex (between the cuticle and the medulla), and the Cuticle (the outermost layer of the hair).

Peppermint Oil - From the peppermint herb, this extremely potent oil is extracted by steam distillation. Peppermint oil has antibacterial, anti-inflammatory, antiviral, insecticidal, antispasmodic, and carminative properties. These properties can relieve a dry scalp while also stimulating hair growth and giving hair a healthy sheen or shine.

pH - is an abbreviation for "potential hydrogen". pH is a scale of 0 (highly acidic) to 14 (highly basic) for ranking the relative acidity or alkalinity of a liquid solution.

Pineappling - The pineapple is basically just gathering your hair to the very top of your head, securing with a loose hair band or a scrunchie, and leaving the ends loose. Pineappling preserves your curls by alleviating the problem of mashing your curls down as you sleep. Since you'll be sleeping on the hair from the nape, the curls at the crown portion of your head will still be intact in the morning.

Plopping - This refers to a technique for drying your hair by placing it into a cloth or t-shirt.

Pre-Poo - is the process to soften the blow of detangling and washing hair. It is an oil or conditioner applied to hair prior to shampooing. Pre-pooing your hair before washing makes hair easier to detangle, but it also keeps hair moisturized as shampooing (especially with a clarifying shampoo) can strip it of necessary oils.

Product Junkie - a natural who compulsively buys hair care products and is always in search of the newest and the best. They cannot pass up a new item from any line and surely go 'all in' on sales.

Protective Styling - are hairstyles that require low maintenance and are considered to be a "break" from daily handling. Hair is usually put up and away to protect from the environmental pollutants, styling and even friction from clothing. The idea is that hair is put away and protected. Popular, protective styles are braids, twists, updos, wearing wigs or weaves, just to name a few.

Quinoa - is called the "miracle" grain. While a tasty superfood, Quinoa is also great for hair by helping to repair damage to the hair shaft. A vegetable protein, Quinoa helps to protect hair by coating and strengthening hair.

Rhassoul Clay - Moroccan clay, aka Rhassoul clay, comes from the Atlas mountains of Morocco. It is packed with minerals and has high absorption for impurities found in hair. It can also help to relieve dryness, flakes in your scalp, and assist with detangling your hair.

Rosehip seed oil - Harvested from the seeds of rose bushes, rosehip oil is is full of vitamins, antioxidants and essential fatty acids. It contains a very high concentration of Vitamin A, which is essential in cell turnover. This means that this remarkable oil helps in the promotion of cell regeneration, healing and cell production. It makes this oil helpful with hair growth and the repair of hair damage.

Rosemary Oil - Very popular in the Mediterranean region as a culinary herb, rosemary oil also has great benefits for hair and scalp. Rosemary oil has anti-fungal properties that aid in dandruff and helps to stimulate hair growth. Many use it as a hair tea.

Safflower Oil - Extracted from the safflower plant, this edible colorless, flavorless and odorless oil has been used for years in helping with thinning hair and baldness. Rich in vitamin E and fatty acids, this is an ideal light oil for low porosity strands. Safflower seed oil is great for growth and can be used in scalp massages as it helps with blood circulation to the hair follicles. It does penetrate the hair shaft somewhat, which makes it a good choice for moisturizing and conditioning.

Scab hair - is an unscientific term to describe the newly grown hair after one stops chemically relaxing the hair. This hair is extremely dry, unruly and many feel it's merely the lingering chemicals finding its way out of the scalp. There is no way to get around scab hair so even doing a BC (Big Chop) is not going to help eliminate it. You having to learn to work with it.

Sealing Ends - is protecting hair (especially the ends) as they are the oldest and most vulnerable to friction, tangles and breakage. You accomplish this by sealing moisture into hair and especially on the ends to combat split ends, dryness and frizz.

Search & Destroy - A trimming technique that is a bit on the time-consuming side but great for the naturals concerned with holding onto as much as as possible. You take small sections of hair (about an inch) and searching for split ends, knots, or frays. Cut about 1/4 above the split end or knot to ensure all the damaged hair is removed. Again, this is time consuming but can be done as often as you like and can be just something you do when watching TV, or whatever. Make sure to use the right shears and to have proper lighting. Many naturals do this in between regulars trims.

Senegalese Twists - A popular protective style, Senegalese twists or "rope twists" are created by wrapping Kanekalon braiding hair around the root of sectioned natural hair. Hair is two-strand twisted to the ends of the hair shaft. They are typically easier to remove than box braids.

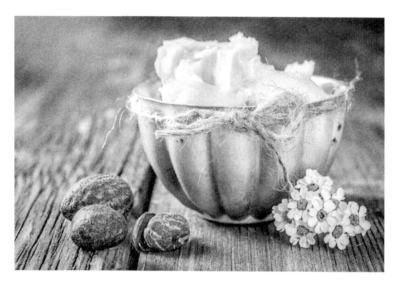

Shea Butter - comes from the nut of the shea tree, and is rich in vitamins A and E. The most popular, widely recognizable Shea butter is produced from the Shea-Karite tree in East and West Africa. Not only does this butter work as an excellent sealant for the hair, it also conditions and softens the hair, as well as protects against harmful UV rays. Unbeknownst to many, Shea butter can also be used to soothe scalp irritation, which happens more often than not during the winter months.

Shingling - is a wash & go styling technique to maintain curl definition. Using a styling curl cream or curl gel, product is liberally applied section-by section to clean, saturated hair. The styling product is applied to small sections of hair and then each section is smoothed between the thumb and forefinger, in a downward motion from root to tip.

Shrinkage - is a term used to describe the reduction of the visual length of hair due to nature; it will "shrink" as it dries. The tighter the curl, coil, or kink, the more shrinkage one will have. When hair is wet, or pulled, the length is apparent. As hair dries, it recoils into its natural texture pattern.

Sisterlocks - were invented by hair expert Dr. JoAnne Cornwell. This patented method of weaving hair into tiny dreadlocks using a specialized tool can only be installed by recognized technicians. Much smaller than traditional locks, this technique allows the small locks to be highly versatile in hairstyling.

SLS - Sodium Laureth Sulfate or Sodium Lauryl Sulfate.

Slip - refers to the slipperiness of a product. These conditioners (regular, leave-in) are are crucial to naturals as they are necessary to detangle tresses productively. Slip makes detangling task easier with less hair being yanked out or in tangles.

Stretched Styles - refers to hairstyles that stretch hair and allow one's true length to be seen without the usage of heat like a flat iron. Styles like roller sets, twist and braid outs are just a few.

Sulfate Free Shampoo - are shampoos free of sulfates or primary surfactants. They are milder detergents that don't completely wash away hair's much needed moisture. Most do not lather and are great for 3 & 4 hair textures or color-treated hair.

Sunflower Seed Oil - Closely related to safflower seed oil, this extremely light oil is extracted from the seeds of the sunflower, which are indigenous to America. A high penetrating oil, right under coconut oil, sunflower oil is an excellent choice for adding moisture to strands, stimulating hair growth and improving scalp health.

Surfactant - are one of many different compounds that make up a detergent. Their function is to break down the combination of water and oils and/or dirt. Sulfates are surfactants but not all surfactants are sulfates.

Tea Tree Oil - is extracted from a tree called Melaleuca alternifolia, which is found in South Wales, Australia. Tea Tree oil is particularly effective against fungus, bacteria and viruses. It also fights dandruff, kills head lice and encourages hair growth by helping to unclog hair follicles and nourish the roots.

Texturizer - is considered a lite relaxer and possess the very same straightening ingredients, either sodium hydroxide (lye) or calcium hydroxide (no-lye). A relaxer completely straightens hair while a texturizer only loosens the curl because it is left on a shorter amount of time. Texturizers are far more successful on shorter hair and even for stylists, it's hard for a texturizer to keep a uniform texture from touch-up to touch-up. This just means some strands may end up completely straight while others may have a curly or wavy pattern. In some cases, the texturizer cannot turn the kinky/coily hair into a curly texture but rather dry damaged hair.

Transitioning - Also called "Long-Term Transitioning," is the term used to describe the act of allowing natural hair to grow out over time while keeping relaxed ends. With this method, chemically treated hair is left intact and trimmed off gradually as your hair grows out. Those of you who don't feel comfortable rocking a short Afro may also find transitioning a better approach to going natural.

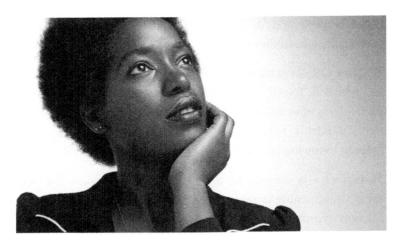

TWA - A Teeny Weeny Afro is what many "going natural" start off with if they choose to Big Chop.

Twist Out - The twist-out is one of the more popular hairstyles that allows for a uniform spiral or coil pattern in one's natural hair. Simply place hair into twists and then unravel for your desired style and this can be achieved on fully wet hair (like right from washday) or on dry hair.

Ucuuba Butter - Another Brazilian tree butter, ucuuba butter has anti-inflammatory and antiseptic properties which is perfect for eczema or any other inflammations that may happen on the scalp. This butter can also help prevent damage from free radicals, and that will improve shine and elasticity which leads to hydrated hair.

Two-Strand Twists - Hair is placed into twists with just two equal sections of parted hair. Different from braiding, two-strands twists are the most popular type of twisting technique for twist outs.

Wash and Go - A method that consists of washing the hair, and applying a leave-in conditioner and styler gel or cream. Adding a styling gel allows hair to dry naturally or you can use a diffuser. Any hair type can achieve a wash and go as each natural rocks their own curl, kink and coil type.

Water-Soluble Silicones - can be penetrated by and dissolved with water, which makes them easier to deal with. The good thing about these silicones is the fact that they don't cause build up, can enhance moisturizing properties, can add humectant qualities, allows moisture penetration, and are easy to remove. It might be beneficial to look into trying out water-soluble silicones if you're hoping to reduce frizz and impart more shine without running the risk of dehydrating your locks.

Water-soluble silicones can be used to straighten the hair and protect the shaft from heat damage, but they will not prevent moisture from penetrating the shaft, which will cause the hair to revert. However, if you are doing the curly-girl method, co-wash regularly, or are prone to dry hair, water-soluble silicones can actually help impart and retain moisture into the hair shaft, making it very curly-friendly.

If you're interested in giving products that contain water soluble ingredients a try, here are the ingredients to look for: PEG-8 (or higher) Dimethicone, PEG-8-PG-coco glucoside dimethicone, Bis-PEG-8 (or higher) Dimethicone, Dimethicone PE-X phosphate, Bis-PEG-8/PEG-8 Dimethicone, Dimethicone copolyol and Bis-PEG-18 methyl ether dimethyl silane.

CHAPTER TEN

PROTECTING YOUR HAIR

The Importance of protecting your hair seems lost on some women who go natural half-heartedly. This is a lifestyle change and while for many, hair is just an accessory, going natural is more than a hairstyle choice and for your natural tresses to thrive, protection MUST be a priority. Here are the top ways to properly protect your hair, and keep it healthy and retain length.

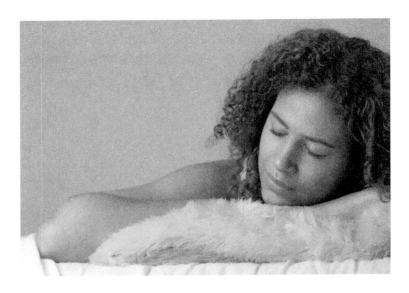

NIGHTTIME ROUTINES

What to do with your natural hair at night is just as important as what to do with it in the morning. While relaxed, we really didn't worry much about it other than making sure to not ruin the style but as we learn more about how to care for our natural tresses, we find the importance of everything we do! When developing a regimen, the same points are pounded into our heads - cleanse, deep condition, moisturize, do protective styles, and etc. But when it comes down to a nighttime routine, we're given general tips, some that aren't really universal.

Caring for your hair as you sleep is just as important as caring for it when you're awake, and even more-so because what you do before bed can be the difference between your curls being on point and being a big, matted mess in the morning. Whether you're rocking a TWA or waist-length locs, it is important to protect your hair as you sleep, in order to retain moisture and preserve your style.

RE-MOISTURIZE & SEAL

If your hair is feeling a bit on the dry side, you'll want to re-moisturize before bed or in the morning. Spritz your hair with a little bit of water or leave-in, and seal with a light oil. If you're rocking a twist/braid out, you can re-twist/braid the hair after sealing, in order to lock in the moisture and decrease the chance of frizzing. If you don't really like spritzing your hair, you can invest in a heat conditioning cap. This is a great option for those with low porosity hair, but also works well for those with medium and high porosity hair.

Less is always more, meaning don't be heavy-handed with resealing. Also realize that moisture comes from very few oils and more from water or water-based products. Slathering heavy oils will not moisturize your hair but rather seal in the moisture you impart. Keeping hair moisturized (whether out or in a protective style) will allow hair to stay healthier as dry, brittle hair is less elastic and more prone to breakage.

HEAT PROTECTANTS

Heat protectants protect your delicate strands from direct heat-styling tools. They are necessary, but far too many Black women haven't been using them or ever heard of them until recently. We as black women have been applying heat to our hair for decades and have been paying a hefty price for it. Many of us have been suffering from heat damage and severe dryness by NOT using heat protectants. Heat protectants can be sprays, lotions or oils that contain silicones to encase the hair and protect it from heat-styling tool. These heat-styling tools are using direct heat and are tools like a flat iron, blow-dryer (without a diffuser) or a flat iron. These tools heat directly touching the hair for drying the hair or straightening the natural curl or coil of the hair texture.

These tools although convenient, are harsh on the hair and dry it out so the much needed moisture our hair needs is depleted. They also create heat damage which is irreversible. We should be using direct heat sparingly (once a month or less) as even one application of direct heat can cause heat damage. If using direct heat make sure to use a heat protectant and preferably one with silicones as silicones create a barrier around the hair to protect it from the heat styling tool.

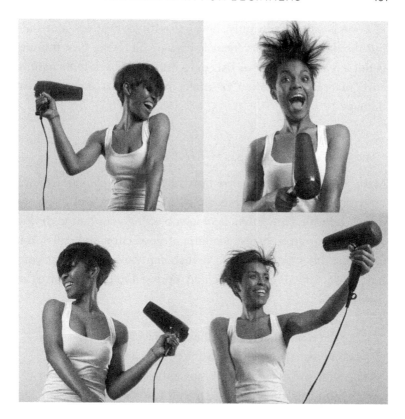

LIMITING HEAT

While there is really nothing wrong with wanting to rock straight hair from time to time, limiting your heat usage is the best way to protect your hair. Heat-styling can dry out hair and even cause you to incur heat damage. Heat damage is irreversible so the best way to deal with it, is to NOT get it. These tools take moisture out of your hair, and while a heat protectant is helpful, what's even better is limiting your heat-styling tool. Never use them daily; even weekly can be too often. Once a month or less is best, so lay off the flat irons, curling wands and blow dryers on hot settings. You can always get straight styles by roller setting and then wrapping hair to get it even straighter.

No one is saying you must never use direct heat on your hair, but the damage you can incur is irreversible. Also, heat training is not a real thing. If your hair does not revert back to its natural curl after an application of direct heat, it has incurred heat damage.

CLOTHING, HEADRESTS & HATS

Many naturals do not realize how often tresses come in contact with our clothing, headrests from car, airplanes and even our own headwear. How often are you subjecting your hair to drying fabrics or furniture that is yanking at your curls and coils? You can limit this type of friction, which can yank or dry out your hair, by a little pre-planning and opting for better choices in headwear.

- Purchase hats with a satin-lining, or wear a satin scarf or bonnet beneath your hat. More brands are creating hats, beanies and even baseball caps with satin linings now.
- Invest in a satin pillowcase as cotton sheets and pillowcases dry out our hair and create friction, which can also create frizz. Buy a couple so you can change them out often.
- Keep hair off shoulders or out of contact from clothing as often as possible. Purse straps, and clothing can yank at hair, create split ends or dry out, especially in colder months.
- This may be over the top, but opt for a satin lining over your car headrest. I have a cheap hat that I turn inside out and cover my headrest so that my hair is not getting frizzy from the cloth headrest in my car.
- Don't just rely on your satin pillowcase for protecting your hair at night. Wear a satin bonnet or scarf at night to further preserve your hairstyle but to also keep hair moisturized while you sleep.

- Take a satin scarf or bonnet on vacay. They are great for airplane flights and whenever you have to use a helmet, if you like doing things that require one.

HEALTHY LIVING

Your hair needs protein, nutrients, and vitamins to grow and remain strong and healthy. The best way to get that into your hair is through healthy eating and living. All the supplements in the world cannot protect hair better than drinking lots of water, exercising and eating right. No pill on the market will ever replace healthy eating and living for optimal hair growth. By eating a balanced meal, exercising, getting enough hours of sleep and drinking enough water, you are not only protecting your hair, but also giving it all it needs to grow strong and look beautiful.

PROTECTIVE HAIRSTYLES

Protective hairstyles require low maintenance and are considered to be a "break" from daily handling. Hair is usually put up and away to protect from the environmental pollutants, styling and even friction from clothing. The idea is for hair to be put away and protected. Popular, protective styles are braids, twists, updos, wearing wigs or weaves but if they are NOT correctly maintained, taken out on time or given time in between for rest, are detrimental to protecting your hair.

Hair still needs to be regularly washed, conditioned and moisturized while in a protective style. You should also give hair a treatment in between these styles. For example, braids or weaves need at least two weeks of rest before another install. Never leave them in longer than they are supposed to be left in and if you are wearing wigs, take them off once you get home to allow the scalp to breathe.

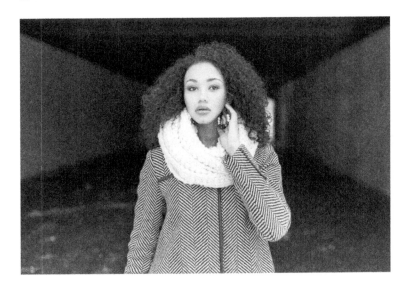

WEATHER

The weather can cause damage to our hair. Sun, wind, environmental pollutants and even the cold are often harsh on our delicate strands. Just as you protect your skin from these elements, you also need to do so with your strands. The sun can burn your scalp and massive hours from the UV in sunlight can significantly alter your hair cuticles and the porosity. You can actually incur dry, brittle hair that's faded and limp from sun damage so protect your hair! Natural oils like Marula and Neem Oil, or even Shea Butter help block those harmful UV rays. You can also always protect your hair and scalp with hats, head wraps and scarves.

During colder months, many naturals suffer from the dryness outside as well as the dryness inside from cranking up the heat to stay warm. Drink a lot of water and consider investing in a humidifier to keep some moisture in the air and your hair.

HANDLING

Less is more when it comes to protecting your hair from your own handling. Even by washing our hair, we can cause damage, so always make sure to condition after every wash day. Make moisturizing a priority and use as little manipulation in your styling. Try not to fiddle with your hair absentmindedly as that can cause breakage and dryness. More manipulation can lead to more damage.

CHAPTER ELEVEN

HAIR TYPES, DENSITY & POROSITY

Hair-typing provides the basis for the type of curls you have. Although it is obvious enough that natural hair varies in texture, hair-typing is a system that makes it easy to point out what category your strands fall into. Hair-typing is a big thing in natural hair and while the verdict is out on whether it truly figures it all out for you, many still subscribe to it in aiding in hair product purchases and how to care for one's own curls.

There is more than just one hair-typing system and while many may favor one over all the others, all bring some very vital information to the table. I've listed a few that you should get to know and you can then figure out which best suits your hair's needs.

HAIR TYPE

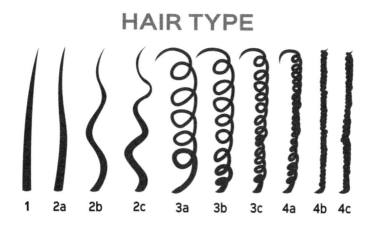

1 2a 2b 2c 3a 3b 3c 4a 4b 4c

HAIR TYPES

Andre Walker Hair-Typing System

Andre Walker divides hair into four categories: type 1- straight hair, type 2- wavy hair, type 3- curly hair and type 4- kinky hair. Each of these categories also have sub-categories that divide them into different segments, depending on texture and curl pattern. This is probably the most popular hair-typing system that most naturals gravitate to.

LOIS Hair-Typing System

This typing system determines hair type depending on its pattern, strand size and texture. If your hair falls in right angles with no obvious curve, it is considered an L. If your hair forms tight curls resembling an O, it is considered as O. If your hair has no bend and lies flat on the head, it is considered an I. If your hair has S-shaped curls, it is considered an S.

Fia's Hair-Typing System

This typing system is an upgraded combination of the two previous ones. It defines hair type using three classifiers: definition of curls, visible moisture content and volume of the hair. The second classifier (moisture content) helps to determine if the hair is Fine - smooth and silky, Medium - a texture between fine and coarse, or Coarse - thick and wiry feeling strands.

Density

When discussing hair types or hair-typing, we have to factor in one's hair density as well. Hair density is simply a measurement of hair's thickness and depends upon the thickness of individual strands as well as the number of strands on your head. Hair density relates to how many strands of hair you have per square inch on your scalp. Knowing your hair's density is helpful for which hair products to use on your hair and which styles will look the best on you as thicker hair will style easier with longer layers and thinner hair will style easier with blunt cuts.

The easiest way to determine your own hair density is to allow your hair to hang loose and look at it in a mirror. If you can see your scalp without moving your hair, then you most like have low density. If you can see your scalp with little or no effort then you most likely have medium density and if it's hard to see your scalp, you have high hair density.

Porosity

Hair porosity is extremely important in hair care, but most just concern themselves with texture. Hair porosity refers to how well your hair absorbs water or moisture, oils and even chemicals like color or straighteners. It affects the strands and health of your hair on many levels. Your hair's porosity will determine how well your hair takes on color, prevents breakage and even get moisture into your strands. Knowing your hair's porosity is necessary to know how certain products, procedures and techniques will effect your hair. I now know I have high porosity (the most damaging of them all).

Low Porosity hair has the hardest time getting moisture, oils and even chemicals in because there is a tightly bound cuticle layer with overlapping scales. What is good about this type is it will hold the moisture in very well once you get it in there.

Medium Porosity hair is the middle of the road and requires the least amount of maintenance of all three. The cuticle layer is less tight and allows just enough moisture in and retains it well.

High Porosity hair can be either inherent or from damage as the strands with this type of hair have gaps and holes in the hair's cuticle. This is often over chemical processing from straighteners or color, or even heat damage. The problem is not getting moisture in but keeping it in as the raised cuticle can receive as much as it can lose.

Width

Hair width is the circumference or thickness of each individual hair strand. They can be coarse (thick and strongest), medium (strands are neither too thick or too thin, but are strong and elastic) or fine (strands have a small circumference and width, are delicate and can incur damage easily). Your hair's width affects your ability to retain length and naturals with coarse or medium hair width can retain it easier than naturals with fine strands. Hair width is extremely important as it plays a major role to strength and how susceptible your strands are to damage.

To find one's hair width, simply hold up a strand to the light. If the strands is so thin, that you almost cannot see it, then you have fine hair. If the strand is easily visible, you have coarse hair and if it is neither too thin or thick, you have medium width.

CHAPTER TWELVE

EVERYTHING YOU NEED TO KNOW ABOUT PROTECTIVE STYLING

Protective Styling is big in the natural hair community. Many women use them for several reasons from versatility, less time doing hair and for the most obvious reason...to protect hair and maximize hair growth. Let's delve into the world of protective styling so you have not just the full picture, but an informative one on why or why not you will take the protective styling plunge.

WHAT IS PROTECTIVE STYLING?

Protective styling is subjective as it can vary from natural to natural but in a nutshell, it is any style that protects your hair from physical, chemical and/or environmental disturbances. A true protective style requires little to no manipulation, protects the ends of hair (the oldest and most fragile parts of the strand) and is put away from manipulation anywhere from a few weeks to a few months. As natural hair evolves, the notion that only a few styles fall into this category is changing. More naturals realize there does not have to be strict guidelines on what and what does NOT constitute as a "protective style."

WHAT ARE PROTECTIVE STYLES?

Technically, protective styles can be any style that keeps your ends out of harm's way. Most people think only certain styles that fall strictly in that category are protective styles but there are several styles that are protective even if your hair is not tucked away in braids, weaves or a tight updo. Here is a list of first the most popular protective styles:

TYPES OF PROTECTIVE STYLES: BRAIDS

Braids are one of the more popular protective styles and fun to rock all year long. The styles are pretty endless and each style has its own timeline for installing and taking down. Here is a list: Box braids, Crochet Braids, Dutch, Fishtail, French, Ghana, Micro, and Milkmaid. Many will add extension hair for volume and/or length. You can install them yourself or enlist the help of a stylist, though price is a factor, especially on the type of hair you choose as you can use synthetic or human hair.

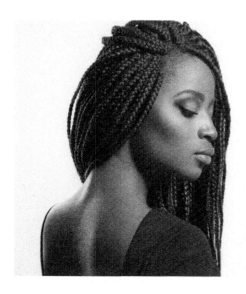

Box - They can be small, medium or large, and short or long. This style can last only up to 12 weeks and should not be left in longer. Hair and scalp can be cleansed while in box braids, and a spritz or braiding spray keeps hair and scalp moisturized.

Crochet Braids - One of the most versatile and popular braids for the last few years is Crochet Braids or Latch hook braids. This style involves crocheting synthetic hair extensions to natural hair with a latch hook or crochet hook. They are quicker to install than other braids so the expense is much cheaper. Crochet braids can stay in anywhere from 4 to 8 weeks, depending on the intricacies of your braid pattern and upkeep.

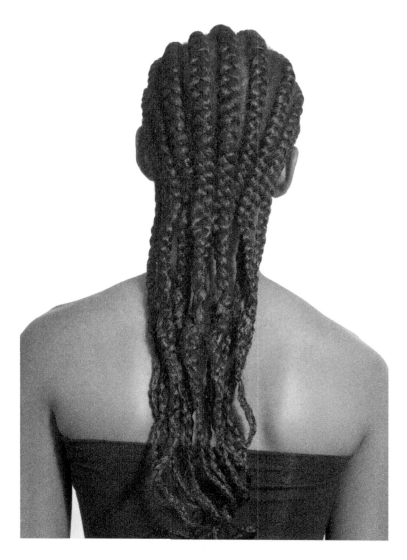

Cornrow - Also, can be small or large and often extension hair is added to give volume and length along with more style options. The larger the cornrow, the shorter time they stay in your hair.

Larger cornrows can stay in about a week and smaller ones can stay in 4 weeks. Hair and scalp can be washed.

Ghana - An African style of braiding, Ghana braids can last for weeks and are extremely versatile. The major difference between Ghana braids and cornrows is the technique. Ghana braids start off with less extension hair in the front for a more natural look and gradually add more hair throughout the braid for a fuller natural look.

Fishtail - There are a few styles under the heading of protective styles that are new to naturals or just not considered a traditional protective style. Fishtails braids are one of them and this highly fashionable take on the french braid is a favorite summer style. Just like a french braid, this style can last up to a week to a week and a half.

Micro - Micros braids are tiny, delicate braids that are tightly woven into hair and are still quite popular for black women to rock. They last a long time and require minimal daily maintenance. They are more suited for shorter hair and the install is long even with short tresses. They should be kept in no longer than 8 weeks but many have gone as long as 12 weeks. Hair must be washed and conditioned regularly with these braids. Also, make sure they are not too tight or you could suffer from breakage, usually around the hairline.

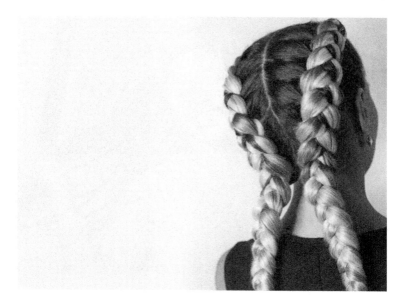

French - French braids or a braid where hair is gathered into one large braid down the back of the head, are similar to fishtail braids and last just as long (around 1 week or slightly longer). They can be done solely on your own hair or with extension hair for fullness and length and can be twisted into elaborate updos for style variations.

Milkmaid - Milkmaid braids (often called halo braids) are simply two pigtail braids that are wrapped on top of your head. The larger the braid the prettier it is, and many add extension hair to create a longer and fuller set of braids to wrap on your head. This style may last up until 1 week or a tad bit longer if the braid was tight (but not too tight), and you cover hair at night to help preserve the style and fight off frizz.

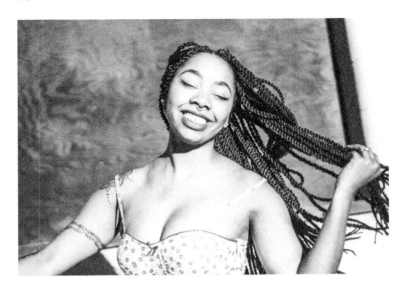

Twists - Twists are another highly popular protective style and often used by naturals since they offer more volume than traditional braids. Twists use a two-strand braiding technique that allows twisted hair to give off a fuller effect (for volume seekers) and extension hair can be added for even more volume and length. Make sure to get hair in tip top shape prior to the install.

Marley - Marley twists, also called Kinky Twists, are two-strand twists created with extension hair known as Marley Braid Hair. They are bigger than Senegalese twists, and this style can be left in for up to 12 weeks.

Havana - Havana twists use Havana hair extensions and are much more expensive than Marley Twists. They are much lighter than Marley twists and have a rougher texture than Marley twists (and fuller and fluffier) and they can last up to 12 weeks just like Marley twists.

Flat - Flat twists require you know how to cornrow, as hair is parted into cornrowed sections and is flat-twisted instead of being braided down the head. Just like cornrows, this style can have extension hair added for fullness and/or length and the style last anywhere from 1 to 4 weeks.

Senegalese - Also called "rope twists," Senegalese twists are created by wrapping Kanekalon braiding hair around the root of your sectioned natural hair. Hair is then two-strand twisted from the root all the way down the length of the hair. These twists have shine and can last anywhere from 8 to 16 weeks with proper upkeep.

Two-strand - Hair is placed into twists with just two equal sections of parted hair. Braiding hair can be added for volume and length. Often used for a twist out, but if left in, this is a protective style as long as the ends are not in contact with clothing and manipulation. Often, naturals will create elaborate updos with this style to make it more protective and last longer. This style can last for up to 2 weeks.

Three-strand - Similar to two-strand twist, this style is created with three individual pieces of hair intertwined around each other to create one twist. This style can also last for up to 2 weeks and considered a protective style if it is not manipulated, in contact with clothing and pinned up.

Mini - Mini twists are tiny twists smaller than a pencil and a great protective style that lasts long (from 3 to 6 weeks) than other twist styles. The install and take down is lengthy, but this style is highly versatile and very popular.

Chunky - Chunky twists are large twist styles that are often created in updos and other protective style. Most often used for twist-outs, when used in a protective style like a high bun or milkmaid version of twists, this style can last anywhere from 1 to 2 weeks.

Faux Locs - An increasingly popular style among naturals, faux locs are meant to look like real dreadlocks. They can be created by using human hair, yarn, or synthetic braiding hair. With proper maintenance, this fun protective style can last up to 12 weeks.

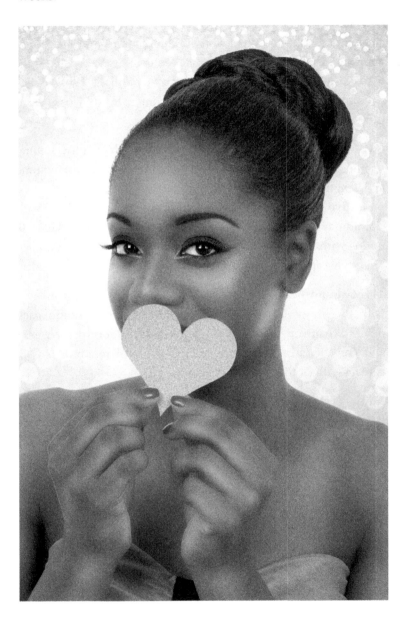

UPDOS

Updos are hairstyles where the hair is swept up and fastened away from the face and neck, and considered elegant. What many newly naturals are unaware of is their functionality as a great protective style. Updos are extremely versatile and are only limited to the creativity of the wearer. From braided high buns to a rope-twisted halo braid, updos are great options for everyday work/school and play. The length of time you can keep hair in this style depends on how intricate it is, and with hair almost always tucked in or braided up ensure you are protecting your hair well.

Popular updos are worn by most natural wearers because they are easy to create buns, chignons, top knots and ninja buns. Remember, adding hair, twists or braids into these styles will create a new and fresh take on them. Even a simple roll and tuck updo is considered a protective style. Never feel you have to spend a lot of money or time on an updo to protect your hair. Many of these styles will add extension hair to give the style a fuller look or create intricate braids or twists in the updo. The sky's the limit, but make sure to protect hair at night with a scarf or bonnet, and know that regularly washings and conditionings are still needed.

WIGS

Wigs are increasingly becoming the ultimate low-stress protective style for women, and that most-certainly includes naturals. Many are opting for rocking wigs when transitioning and while this style allows for mega versatility, adhering to a few rules will allow this style to actually protect. Here are a few tips that need to be implemented so that wig life is positive.

Wash Your Hair Regularly - This may seem like a no-brainer, but keeping your own hair and scalp clean while wearing a wig is very important. Since your scalp is covered for the majority of the day, there's a chance that sweat has been accumulating, which can cause an unpleasant smell. Co-wash your hair weekly in order to rid the scalp of any sweat and dead skin that has started to build up, even if you choose not to wash with shampoo that often.

Moisturize, Moisturize, & Moisturize Some More - Wig caps can suck the moisture right out of your hair, so remember to moisturize the hair multiple times per week. Once you finally get home, take the wig cap off, lightly spritz your hair with some water or a liquid leave-in and pat it into the hair. Don't wet the hair too much; just spritz enough water to replenish some moisture into your strands. Make sure to NEVER place a wig on damp or wet hair!

Detangle and braid up the hair - If your hair is long enough to get tangled, you need to make sure it is detangled and braided down before applying your wig cap. Not only does this reduce the look of bumps under your wig, but it will prevent the hair from becoming matted by the friction of it against the wig cap.

Massage & Care For Your Scalp - Neglecting your scalp while wearing a wig is the worst thing you can do. Dry scalp and severe dandruff are two side effects of regular wig-wearing that is the easiest to contract. Apply anti-fungal oils such as tea tree mixed with carrier oils for scalp massages.

Rocking wigs as a protective style is as great way to keep hair healthy and moisturized. Make sure you care for your hair underneath and watch it thrive. Do not become too dependent on the wigs as you still need to learn how to care and style your own hair.

Weaves - Weaves are a form of hair extensions that are woven or glued, into the hair from a track. Many women are leaving the glues alone as they can suffocate the scalp and cause breakage from the roots. I don't also recommend becoming too dependent on weaves as you will become an expert on the weave and not one on your own natural hair. Weaves are great as a PS, as long as you give your hair a breather between installs and don't have them in too long or too tight, but far too many women are relying on them for too long and finding that they cannot live without them. Use this method but change it up from time to time and give your own hair a chance to get some air. Most importantly, allow yourself the opportunity to learn how to care for your natural strands.

DO PROTECTIVE STYLE REALLY WORK?

Yes, and no. Yes, protective styles do fully protect your hair but if you are not still maintaining a healthy lifestyle for your hair, the protective style will not work and could even damage your hair. If you make caring for your hair your first priority, then yes, that protective style will work well.

Is Protective Styling the ONLY way to grow long hair?

Not at all. There are plenty of women rocking long natural hair who have never tried a protective style a day in their life! It's not the "be all for everyone. While many (and I do mean, many) swear by them, protective styling may not be attractive to all women going natural who want long hair. Some women have found their hair to grow stronger and longer while in a PS 90% of the time and they make sure to do everything right for their hair while in them. Others have found the same results without using a PS. It is up to the woman to determine if she wants to try it out and see if her growth made a major increase while fully protected. There are tons of protective styles to choose from. Changing them up can keep a PS from becoming boring, if you feel your hair needs that extra protection for optimal growth. Whether you opt for a PS or not, we all need to protect our hair from the elements, heat-styling tools, our clothing and even the sun, so you will need to determine how much protecting your strands need to thrive.

CRUCIAL TIPS FOR SUCCESSFUL PROTECTIVE STYLING

Just like anything else, there are necessary steps to ensure your protective style works properly, does not cause damage and looks amazing while your natural hair is in the style.

- Give hair at least two weeks in between installs for

braids, weaves and some twisted styles. Hair needs a break to breathe and enjoy the lack of tension.

- Make sure to properly cleanse, condition and fully detangle hair prior to placing hair into a protective style. Hair will be up in that style for at least a few days on up to a few months and hair needs to be fully ready for the task at hand. Never install a protective style on dirty hair or hair that hasn't been properly detangled. You can end up with sour or dirty hair, or a mass of knots too hard to fix after you take it down.

- Deep condition too! You should be doing a DC on every wash day as it protects and prepares hair for styling. If unable to DC, make it a priority before the protective so it can handle all the styling that comes with creating the look.

- Get a trim, if needed. Those ends need to be protected, but make sure they are strong and not splitting or the protective style will not be protecting anything good.

- Expect a lot of shedding when you take out your PS. We can shed up to 100 hairs a days. So, if you hair has been in a PS for two months, all that shed hair is just waiting to come out. Don't panic as this is normal, but don't yank out the good hairs with the bad ones. Take your time taking down your style, so that you are only removing the snags, tangles and shed hairs.

- Give hair a protein or moisturizing treatment in-between installs of the PS. Hair in a protective style has been pinned up, covered or in tension for a period of time. For the longer PS, give hair a much needed treatment to make sure your hair stays damage free and beefed up for health. This is the time to pamper your hair, so it stays strong.

- Never leave hair in a PS longer than recommended. You run the risk of hair locking up, breaking off or worse. Yes, some of these styles are expensive and you want to get your monies worth, but if you have to sacrifice the health of your hair to save a few dollars, then the PS is really not for you.

- Make sure your PS is not too tight! A PS that is too tight runs the risk of breaking the most fragile hairs, like along the hairline. Keep in mind that it should never give you massive headaches.

- Wash your synthetic hair before installing your PS. Soaking some synthetic hair like Kanekalon Hair in Apple Cider Vinegar removes the coating sprayed on the hair. Many women have bad allergic reactions to this coating like bumps, scalp irritations or worse. A lot of braiding hair brands have this coating and it is not necessary to keep on the hair for you to keep your style.

- Put in the proper time and effort for the Protective Style you choose. Some Protective Styles are pretty simple to care for while others need more work. Make sure you know exactly what is expected of you so that your style lasts longer and remains damage free to your strands.

CHAPTER THIRTEEN

HOW TO GET MAXIMUM HAIR GROWTH!

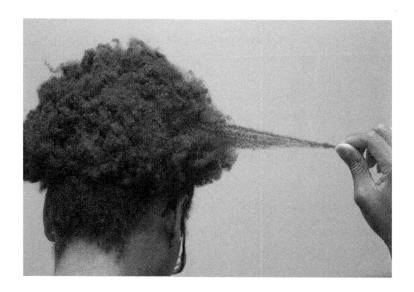

Let's face it...most of us want to grow hair faster, longer and bigger, and in the shortest amount of time necessary. While our hair shrinks and looks shorter than it really is, our hair is forever growing and getting longer. What many of us really want when we say we want maximum growth is length retention. Length retention is keeping the oldest hair on our head as long as possible and not subject to breakage. Here is a list of the best ways to get optimal growth but also keep those older strands longer by protecting them.

EVENING SCALP MASSAGES

Everyone wants to have long, healthy hair. One of the easiest ways to achieve that can be done at night with a simple scalp massage. Scalp massages (with or without oil) can increase blood circulation to the hair follicles and condition the scalp, all while boosting the strength of the hair roots.

You just use your fingertips with or without a light oil and massage gently in a circular motion. Great oils for scalp massages are coconut, olive, jojoba, lavender or rosemary. You can blend some too. I love using jojoba oil with a drop or two of lavender since lavender is excellent at aiding a dry, flaky scalp and has anti-inflammatory, antiseptic, and analgesic properties. A few nights a week is all you need. If you are interested in doing the job quicker and more effectively, then you may want to try a generic scalp massaging shampoo brush to help with the process. They work wonders and are reasonably priced.

ESTABLISH A SOLID HAIR CARE REGIMEN

One of the common denominators that many successful Naturals point to as critical component in their hair's growth factor is a consistent hair care regimen. Examples of a regular hair washing regimen might include but is not limited to any of the following:

- Pre-Poo then wash hair every week with a moisture-rich shampoo and deep conditioner or;
- Wash hair every week with a moisture-rich shampoo, plus use of a deep conditioner, and alternate each week with a protein treatment or;

- Wash hair every week with a moisture-rich shampoo and conditioner, and alternate every other week with a deep conditioner.

Regardless of the hair care regimen you establish, pay attention to how your hair responds to the regimen and products you use. Be sure to adjust periodically. Some natural divas find that using a co-wash in between shampoos works well while others periodically use clarifying shampoos to remove product buildup.

Next, know your hair oils and which oils work best for your hair type. Did you know that certain hair types respond differently to certain oils? Your oil choices can have a significant impact on how much moisture your hair retains as well as the degree of shine visible in your hair.

Get trims regularly. Not as often as you did when relaxed, but when it is necessary. Ask a natural hair stylist if you do not know how often to go. The less manipulation and chemicals you place in your hair, the less often you need a trim.

KEEP HAIR & SCALP CLEAN

Hair grows out of the scalp. If you are suffering from clogged hair follicles, inadequate or too much sebum production or product build-up, you are hindering your hair from growing at its peak. Exfoliating the scalp helps remove dead skin cells and unclog pores. This is important when dealing with a flaky scalp, build-up, stunted hair growth or improper sebum production. While all of these characteristics should be checked out by your dermatologist, exfoliating the scalp can help in the meantime. Scalp exfoliation has been known to help with scalp conditions such as psoriasis or eczema, promote healthy hair growth and even reduce shedding.

EAT WELL

There are certain foods that will help hair grow as fast as possible like foods full of fatty acids and proteins. Lean fish, leafy green veggies, seeds and beans are all great examples of foods that our hair needs for full growth support. Stay on top of your hair growth game by eating foods full of vitamins A, B, C, and E, iron, copper, magnesium selenium and zinc.

TAKE SUPPLEMENTS

Nothing beats a well-balanced meal to get the essential vitamins we need for healthy bodies and hair, but too many of us do not eat as well as we should. This can hinder us from getting all the vitamins we need for optimal hair growth. Couple that with the fact that most women will suffer with some form of hair thinning in their lives. You can see why hair vitamins are extremely popular in the beauty community.

There are plenty of vitamins on the market, so you have to do your homework. Hair vitamins are just one way to get the daily dose of those vital nutrients that aid in stronger hair, for a longer retention on our heads!

HAVE A NIGHTTIME ROUTINE

No matter the products you use, how many supplements you take or how much water you drink, if you do not have a great nighttime routine, you are doing more harm good. While you sleep, your hair can tangle, which promotes breakage. Cotton pillowcases also cause your hair to catch, twist, and break as you toss and turn throughout the night. Satin or silk pillowcases or satin bonnets have much finer textures that are smoother against the hair strands and won't whisk away moisture or create frizz.

A great nighttime routine will save styles and save hair. Whether you need to re-twist or simply give yourself a much needed scalp massage, make sure your routine is more than you just flopping down on a cotton pillowcase and being sorry in the morning.

LIMIT OR REMOVE HEAT-STYLING

Heat-styling is a big contributor to limiting one's hair growth. They can cause dehydration of your strands, rapid water loss, protein damage and oxidation of pigment particles, according to Tonya McKay, polymer scientist and cosmetic chemist. Direct heat (curling irons, flat irons or blow dryers without diffusers) can create heat damage.

Heat damage is excessively high heat permanently breaking the S-S or disulfide bonds within the hair strands. Those bonds give hair its strength along with protein cross-links and when damaged, they cannot be repaired. Heat damage is irreversible. Natural hair should be steering clear of heat or using sparingly. When using heat, always use a heat protectant but don't expect a protectant to be your savior. Use the lowest setting when heat-styling, and do not use it often.

STEER CLEAR OF CRASH DIETS

Using extreme measures like crash dieting doesn't just negatively affect your health. It may cause hair loss. Dietary factors affect all phases of hair growth and when you are not getting enough nutrients (most common in crash diets) you can cause your hair to grow at a slower pace or even create hair fall or loss. If you want to lose weight, do it the right way by eating well balanced meals so you are not hurting your body or hair growth.

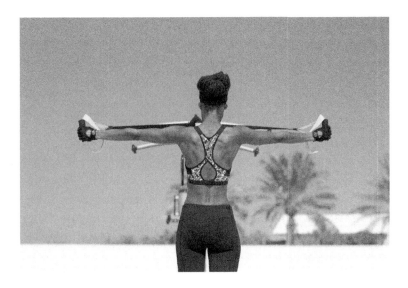

STAY HEALTHY

No one says you need to be running marathons, but staying healthy is crucial to healthy hair growth. Many illnesses will negatively affect your hair growth. Hormonal changes, medical conditions and even some medicines can affect your hair's growth or even cause hair loss.

According to a recent study, Women who have been ill or taking medicine are 81% more likely to suffer from hair loss and thinning than those who have not. Over half (58%) of women who have been ill or taking medicine are experiencing signs of hair loss.

ENLIST THE HELP OF THE THREE C'S

Caffeine, Cayenne and Cinnamon. These three items are by far the cheapest, easiest to get and hard-working hair loss remedies found right in your very kitchen! Not always considered for hair, these substances all have proven growth properties that aid in hair loss problems. Let's get started on learning what they are, what they do and how you can use them to gain longer and stronger tresses.

Caffeine. Whether you love coffee, tea or even soda, caffeine is what gives you that jolt and has you craving for more. This substance stimulates our Central Nervous System and can be found in over 60 plants. The biggest benefit caffeine brings to hair is to improve hair growth and structure. Caffeine stimulates and interacts with the hair follicles. It even regulates hair growth so it can promote it and thwart hair loss. You can just keep drinking your morning cup of Joe to gain that benefit or you can take it a step further (like I do) and enlist in a coffee rinse from time to time to help with shedding hair.

Caffeine must be applied directly to hair for this benefit (through coffee or tea), which adds shine as well as depth to dark hair. Great for hair butters or conditioners to just add to them to increase hair's natural sheen or shine that many naturals complain their hair is lacking. Just brew a strong cup of coffee, espresso or black tea (all three are great hair loss remedies) and allow to cool. Pour over your head after you wash and condition. Leave in for 20 minutes and then rinse out.

Cayenne. One of the spicier hair loss remedies, Cayenne or Cayenne pepper, hot chili pepper in the Capsicum family, originated in Central and South America. Cayenne peppers are closely related to bell peppers and jalapeños. They have been and are still a popular spice used in many different regional styles of cooking, and have been used medicinally for thousands of years.

Cayenne pepper has anti-inflammatory, anti-allergen, anti-fungal and anti-irritant properties. It contains vitamin A, vitamin B6, vitamin C, beta-carotene, manganese and potassium. While all are amazing for our bodies, these properties are great for stopping hair loss and promoting hair growth. In a nutshell, it's the capsaicin in cayenne pepper that stimulates hair growth by stimulating blood circulation to the hair follicles, which ensures better nutrition along with healthier hair growth. Capsaicin also stimulates dormant hair follicles, thus helping hair volume and thickness. If that's not enough, it can even add some sheen and softness to your tresses. A cayenne hair mask will strengthen the hair follicles, speed up hair growth, reduce hair loss, eliminate dandruff and seborrhea and normalize the cell renewal process of the scalp. Just be careful when using it.

Cinnamon. There are hundreds of types of cinnamon but only four varieties are used for commercial purposes. The main variety is Cassia Cinnamon which is mainly used in the US and Canada. The second most popular variety of cinnamon is Ceylon Cinnamon which is mostly used in Europe, Mexico and various parts of Asia. You can also find many woman in the natural hair community who swear by cinnamon as of of their favorite hair loss remedies.

Cinnamon contains volatile oils, such as eugenol and trans-cinnamic acid. They have anti-fungal, anti-viral and antioxidant properties. Cinnamon is believed to increase circulation of the scalp. Regular use in a hair mask with strengthen hair follicles, reduces frizz and curtail hair breakage.

PROTECT YOUR HAIR

Whether you enlist the help of a PS or simply do everything to protect your ends without one, protecting your hair is just as important for maximizing your hair growth as keeping it moisturized. The older hair stays longer when you protect them, keep them moisturized, sealed and trimmed. Trim off the raggedy ends before they begin to split. This is how you stave off breakage and allow hair to stay on your head longer.

CHAPTER FOURTEEN

POPULAR INGREDIENTS IN HAIR PRODUCTS YOU MAY NOT KNOW YOUR HAIR

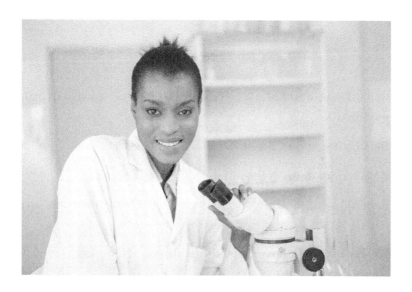

It's hard to learn EVERYTHING about going natural. One of the hardest things to stay on top of is the ingredients we find in our products. Not every ingredient is easy to decipher since many are listed using chemical names and can be misleading. With all my years of blogging and freelance writing, I've had to research ingredients so I can explain what they are and what they can do.

I started creating a list of popular ingredients you would find in natural hair products and as the list grew, I became aware of just how important this type of list could be to all naturals and wanted to share this list with you! I've never shared this list ANYWHERE so you have an edge over other naturals! This is by far not all the ingredients you will find in hair products, but they are the most popular ones that are hard to pronounce and may be unfamiliar to you.

A

Aloe Barbadensis: Aloe vera

Aminomethyl Propanol: pH level adjuster

Amodimethicone: Silicone

B

Behenalkonium Chloride: Essential fatty acid (assist in hair growth)

Behentrimonium Chloride: Conditioning agent

Behentrimonium Methosulfate: Mild hair detangler

Behenyl Alcohol: Fatty alcohol (emollients that soften skin and hair)

Bis-Hydroxy/Methoxy Amodimethicone: Non-water soluble silicone

Bisamino PEG/PPG 41/3 Aminoethyl PG Propyl Dimethicone: Silicone

Butylene Glycol: Humectant

Butyrospermum Parkii: Shea butter

. . .

C

C12-15 Alkyl Benzoate: Emollient esters, provides soft, smooth feel to hair

C13-14 Isoparaffin: Emollient and thickening agent

Caprylic/Capric Triglyceride: Derived from coconut oil and glycerin, emollient)

Cetrimonium Chloride: QUAT, prevent static and build-up in the hair.

Cetearyl Alcohol: Fatty alcohol (emollients that soften skin and hair)

Cetearyl Glucoside: Emulsifier

Cetyl Alcohol: emollient, emulsifier, thickener

Cetyl Dimethicone: Non-water soluble silicone (considered a bad one for hair.)

Cetyl Triethylmonium Olivate Dimethicone PEG-8 Succinate: Silicone derivative of olive oil

Caprylic/Capric Triglyceride: Fatty alcohol (emollients that soften skin and hair)

Ceteareth-20: Emollient and emulsifier

Cetrimonium Chloride: Emulsifying or conditioning agents

Cetrimonium Methosulfate: Surfactant - Emulsifying agent

Cetyl alcohol: Fatty alcohol (emollients that soften skin and hair)

Cetyl esters: Lubricant

Cocamidopropyl Betaine: Foam booster, derived from coconut oil

Cocos Nucifera: Coconut Oil

Cyclopentasiloxane: Conditioner, increases slip

Cyclotetrasiloxane: Makes hair dry quicker

Cyclomethicone: Silicone

D

Decyl Glucoside: Mild non-ionic surfactant

Dicetyldimonium Chloride: Anti-static agent. Prevents flyaways

Dimethicone: Popular Silicone (water-soluble)

Dimethicone Copolyol: Silicone (water-soluble)

Disodium cocamphodiacetate: Mild cleanser made from coconut oil

Distearoylethyl Dimonium Chloride: Hair conditioning antistatic

Distearyldimonium Chloride: Moisturizing and smoothing properties

E

Ethoxydiglycol Oleate: Emollient

G

Glyceryl Stearate: Oil-in-Water emulsifier

Glycol Distearate: Increases the thickness or viscosity

H

Helianthus Annuus: Sunflower seed oil

Hyaluronic Acid: Powerful humectant

Hydrogenated Starch Hydrolysate: Humectant

Hydrolyzed Collagen: Humectant

Hydroxpropyl Starch Phosphate: Naturally derived sugar – emulsifier

I

Isodecyl neopentanoate: Emollient

Isopropyl palmitate: Palm oil based emollient

Isostearamidopropyl Morpholine Lactate: Inhibits the buildup of static electricity

L

Lauramidopropyl Betaine: Surfactant

Laurtrimonium Chloride: Hair conditioning agent

M

Mangifera Indica: Mango seed butter

Methyl Gluceth-10: Humectant

Myristamine Oxide: Foam boosters / surfactants

Myristyl alcohol: Fatty alcohol (emollients that soften skin and hair)

· · ·

N

Neopentyl Glycol Diheptanoatea: Emollient and viscosity increasing agent

O

Olea Europaea: Olive fruit oil

Oleth-20: Oily liquid used to keep the product from separation

P

Panthenol: Humectant with ability to hold moisture

PEG-12 Dimethicone: Silicone based polymer

Peg/Ppg-17/18 Dimethicone: Surfactant, emulsifier

PEG-60 almond glycerides: Fatty acid from almond oil, emollient

PEG-150 Distearate: Emulsifier

Phenoxyethanol: Preservative to inhibit the growth of bacteria

Phenyl Trimethicone: Silicone

Polyacrylamide: Polymer, helps hair hold style

Polyquaternium-4: High curl retention

Polyquaternium-7: Anti-static agent and film former

Polyquaternium-10: Increasing hair body

Polyquaternium 11: Allows hair to hold its style

Polyquaternium-37: Anti-static agent and film former

Polyquaternium-69: Provides hold, increases shine

Polysorbate 20: Emulsifier

Polysorbate 60: Emulsifier

Polysorbate 80: Emulsifier

Potassium Chloride: Viscosity increasing agent

PPG-2 Hydroxyethyl Coco/Isostearamide: Anti-static agent

PPG-10 Cetyl Ether: Emollient

PPG-1 TRIDECETH-6: Emollient and keeps product from separating

Propanediol: Preservative-boosting humectant

Propylene Glycol: Highly effective humectant

Prunus Amygdalus Dulcis: Sweet almond oil

PVP: Fixative, film-former

Q

Quaternium-26: Derivatives of mink oil, hair conditioning agent.

Quaternium-90 Bentonite: Dispersing agent-non surfactant

Quaternium-91: quaternary ammonium salt - keeps hair from fading

R

Retinyl Palmitate: Hair conditioning agent

Ricinus Communis: Castor seed oil

S

SD Alcohol 39-C: Antifoaming agents

Sorbitol: Humectant

Sodium C14-16 Olefin Sulfonate: (harsh cleansing agent) sulfate

Sodium Cocoamphopropionate: Hair conditioning agent

Sodium Cocyl Isethionate: Surfactant from fatty acids in coconut oil

Sodium Methyl Cocoyl Taurate: Mild, anionic, vegetable oil (coconut oil)

Stearalkonium Chloride: Coconut derived emulsifier

Stearamidopropyl dimethylamine: replacement for silicones & adds slip

Stearamidopropyl Dimethylamine: replacement for silicones – water soluble and derived from vegetable oil

Stearyl alcohol: Fatty alcohol

Sucrose: Humectant

T

Tocopheryl Acetate: A form of vitamin E

Trideceth-5: surfactant, emulsifying agent

Dear reader,

We hope you enjoyed reading *Natural Hair For Beginners*. Please take a moment to leave a review in Amazon, even if it's a short one. Your opinion is important to us.

Discover more books by Sabrina R Perkins at

https://www.nextchapter.pub/authors/sabrina-perkins

Want to know when one of our books is free or discounted for Kindle? Join the newsletter at http://eepurl.com/bqqB3H

Best regards,

Sabrina R Perkins and the Next Chapter Team

Printed in Great Britain
by Amazon

18542485R00089